SMILE

Be True to Your Teeth and They'll Never be False to You

By Dr. Robert S. Rauch

THIS BOOK IS DEDICATED
TO THE MEMORY OF
HELEN RAUCH

MOM,

> *Thank you for your warmth, your care,*
> *and your unending love.*
> *Thank you for your guidance and your friendship*
> *that I continually think of.*
> *But most of all, thank you for a legacy*
> *that I will always treasure,*
> *The gift of watching your great smile*
> *fill the world with pleasure.*

D1214892

Acknowledgements

I would like to thank the following people for their contributions to this project. Their comments, additions and deletions are greatly appreciated:

Dr. Andrew M. Barkin   Richard A. Barkin, D.D.S.
Dr. Douglas Barkin   Dr. John C. Britz
Marion Cochran   Tina DeMarco
Dr. Thomas DeGennaro   Clotilde Dudley, R.D.H., M.P.A.
Richard Donahue   Dominic DiBlasi
John F. Gell, D.M.D.   Dr. David M. Knaus
Dr. Robert F. C. LaRosa   Joanne Lewis
Rick Manning   Ira R. Parker, D.D.S., M.P.H.
Dr. Arthur A. Neckritz   Cyrus Settineri
Michael A. Spagnoli, D.C.   Roger G. Reckis, D.D.S.
Richard W. Reddy, D.D.S.   Michael Rotter, D.D.S.
Joseph Woyciesjes, Jr.   Joseph T. Zuaro, D.D.S.

Drawings, artwork, and diagrams are from the pens of
Stephen Zuraw, Howard L. Rauch and Dennis Greenblatt.

Special thanks to:
Herman R. Rauch, Stephen Zuraw and Bette Zuraw.

Extra–Special Thanks to:
My wife Diana and my children, Lauren, Michael and Bryan for their Love, Support and Smiles.

* **ISBN 0–9624076–0–7**

Table of Contents

Introduction

Dentistry is a multi–billion dollar industry. Unfortunately, millions of dollars are wasted each year on incomplete dental health care. This will continue unless the general public is informed about the basics of dental diseases. The causes of dental destruction must be made totally clear to the patient. Only when this has been accomplished can therapy be instituted to effectively cure the disease.

This book clearly illustrates the causes and cures of most dental problems. The vocabulary, drawings and photographs make for enjoyable and informative reading. This will be a home reference that can be used by the entire family.

I want children, adults and seniors to enjoy the benefits of healthy teeth and gums. Effective chewing and confident smiles will promote improved physical and psychological health. These are some of my goals for writing this book.

Today's viewpoint of dental health may change tomorrow. The ideas presented within contain my present personal educated viewpoint of dentistry. **You** are responsible for your dental health, and your dentist should be consulted prior to any change in your dental health care routines.

Accept my gift of education and let everyone take one step closer to a planet filled with healthy smiles.

Dr. Robert S. Rauch, DDS.

"I am convinced that it is of primordial importance to learn more every year than the year before. After all, what is education but a process by which a person begins to learn how to learn."
- Peter Ustinov

CHAPTER 1

Teeth Before Birth

"The future enters into us in order to transform itself in us,
long before it happens."
R.M. Rilke 1875-1926

While mother-to-be undergoes the miraculous event of pregnancy, the child enjoys the warmth and comfort of the womb. Nestled within the mother's inner sanctum, the infant develops at an incredible pace. Eight weeks after conception, the fetus is one inch long. Already many physical characteristics can be seen. Eyes, ears, hands and feet can be clearly defined. At eight weeks in-utero, the first teeth begin to develop. For the next seven months, these teeth will continue to develop. The ultimate strength and structure of these developing teeth is partly determined by the combined chromosomes (genes) of the mother and father.

Because we know that the development of the baby's teeth is ongoing throughout pregnancy, we should consider ways in which we can aid in allowing the oral tissues to develop to their fullest potential. There are several simple, risk-free procedures that will add to better development of your child's teeth.

Vitamins

Take the multi-vitamins that your obstetrician recommends. Vitamins may play an important role in healthy tissue development. Vitamin D is especially helpful to aid in the absorption of calcium from the intestines. Calcium is needed for strong tooth development.

Minerals

Take mineral supplements if your obstetrician recommends them. Minerals comprise an important part of the inorganic tooth structure. The more min-

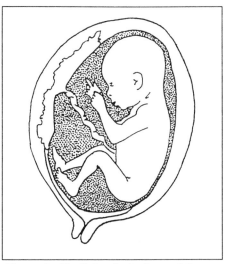

Figure 1 - Teeth begin to form at 8 weeks in-utero.

eral content within the tooth, the stronger the tooth, and the less chance of decay.

Fluoride

Fluoride is a natural mineral that can be incorporated into the developing tooth structure to make the tooth more resistant to decay. The water in your town should be fluoridated for the dental protection of the entire community. One part per million is the present recommended fluoride level in drinking water. Check with your dentist to see whether or not your community's water is fluoridated.

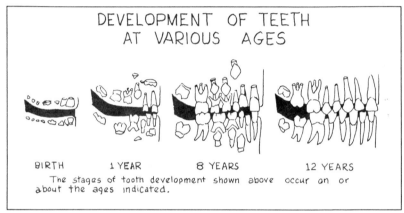

DEVELOPMENT OF TEETH AT VARIOUS AGES

BIRTH 1 YEAR 8 YEARS 12 YEARS

The stages of tooth development shown above occur on or about the ages indicated.

Figure 2 - Development of the teeth.

Reduce emotional stress.

Emotional stress releases adrenaline and other enzymes into the mother's bloodstream. These enzymes can affect the developing child, physically as well as mentally. Researchers have found that high degrees of stress in pregnant mothers yielded children of smaller than average size. Other research has shown that anxiety decreases a pregnant women's ability to absorb certain necessary vitamins. Remember, vitamins and minerals are important for proper child development.

Avoid traumatic injuries to the fetus.

As obvious as it may sound, accidents may cause improper fetal development. If you are pregnant, re-evaluate your physical environment and try to avoid potential danger areas. Even though the developing fetus is in one of nature's most well protected envelopes, extra care should be taken by the expectant mother to avoid physical injury.

Drugs and excessive amounts of alcohol should not be consumed during pregnancy. You do not want your child's growing tissue to look for nourishment in substances that have no constructive value. It is also possible that these substances destroy the vitamins that your child needs.

Rinse, brush and floss your teeth.

Your oral environment is undergoing many changes during pregnancy. Proper rinsing with a pre–rinse, brushing and flossing will limit the possible detrimental effects pregnancy has on your own teeth and gums. Establish good oral care now and your children will learn from you.

Visit your dentist for a professional cleaning while you are pregnant.

This will help you to maintain healthy gum tissue throughout your pregnancy. The pregnant mother's gum tissues often over-react to the presence of plaque. Red irritations and bleeding gums are often a sign of gum inflammation. Early detection and treatment of dental problems will help to maintain the health of your teeth and gums.

Inform the dentist that you are pregnant.

If x-rays are absolutely necessary, make sure that a lead apron is placed over your body. This will lessen any danger of radiation to the fetus. Lead shields should always be used when having dental x-rays whether or not you are pregnant. X-ray paralleling devices, long cones and fast film should also be used by the dentist to decrease radiation exposure.

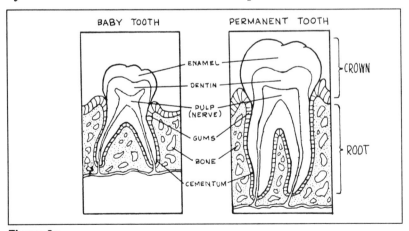

Figure 2a

CHAPTER 2

Birth to Teething

"Give a little love and you get a great deal back."
John Ruskin 1866

Birth is certainly the most miraculous event anyone can witness. As my two children, Lauren and Michael were being lifted skyward, my wife Diana and I knew that we would do anything for their health and safety. They were God's special gifts to Diana and I. Our responsibility as parents had become the priority of our lives together from conception on. Even though I am not suggesting such a moral commitment for everyone, I think parents should try to protect their new child as best they can from any physical danger.

Physical danger to the child's developing dentition (teeth) can be prevented in the first year by these simple procedures:

Breast-feed your child for as long as possible. The colostrum that the child receives from mother's breasts is important. Colostrum is a fluid that precedes the mother's milk. It has high levels of protein, vitamin A and E, along with infection preventing antibodies for the newborn child.

If the baby develops symptoms of constant crying and irritability generally associated with colic, (while breast feeding) eliminate milk and its by-products from your diet. This may lesson baby's abdominal pain. Colic usually clears up between three and five months of age.

If you find problems with breast-feeding, call your local LeLeche League.

If they aren't listed in the telephone book, contact your hospital for assistance in locating them. The LeLeche League can offer invaluable insights and problem solving techniques for a newly nursing mother.

Take the vitamins that your obstetrician recommends. Try to maintain a well balanced diet. Most of your vitamin and mineral needs can be obtained from comprehensive nutritional eating habits along with vitamin supplements.

Give your child the multi-vitamins that your pediatrician recommends.

If your drinking water is not fluoridated, be certain to inform your pediatrician. He/she will prescribe fluoridated vitamins for the baby. Fluoride is a mineral which adds to the strength of the developing tooth, making it more resistant to decay.

RECOMENDED FLUORIDE DOSAGES		
AGE	MGS. (MILIGRAMS) OF FLUORIDE PER DAY	1PPM FLUORIDATED WATER EQUIVALENT
2 WKS- 2 YRS	0.25 MG. =	8 OZ. WATER (1 CUP)
2 YRS- 3 YRS	0.50 MG. =	16 OZ. WATER (2 CUPS)
3 YRS- 16 YRS	1.00 MG. =	32 OZ. WATER (4 CUPS)
FLUORIDE SUPPLIMENTATION SHOULD BE CONSIDERED IF YOUR FAMILY IS NOT DRINKING FLUORIDATED WATER.		

Figure 3

If teeth are present, breast milk residue should be removed from the baby's teeth. Plaque and subsequent decay can begin at this time if the oral environment is not kept clean. Wipe the baby's teeth gently with a gauze pad to clean them.

If a pacifier seems needed, use one that is bio-mechanically designed.

These are less harmful to the developing teeth and jaw relationship than thumbsucking. When the time comes to stop these habits, it is easier to remove the pacifier than it is to remove the thumb.

Thumbsucking, finger-biting, etc. may cause orthodontic problems.

Babies need the stimulation and pleasure derived from the act of sucking. However, there is a point in time when this act can become a psychological habit as opposed to natural stimulation. Past the age of four, strong efforts should be directed at ending these potentially destructive habits. If necessary, consult your dentist for assistance. Your dentist can give you proper information.

Rinse, brush and floss your teeth in front of your child when possible.

The young impressionable child is very observant. Watching parents perform good dental hygiene will act as a foundation for the child's future dental care.

Do not put the baby to sleep with a bottle (Baby Bottle Syndrome).

Night feeding allows milk and juice to interact with bacteria throughout the entire evening and may lead to destruction of the developing dentition. If absolutely necessary a bottle filled with water can be used for night pacification.

If your child has a medical/dental handicap...

If your child has a medical/dental handicap, i.e. cleft palate, there are certain teams of physicians and dentists connected with larger hospitals who can be of great service to you and your child. Early diagnosis and directive therapy will often lessen the amount and severity of future problems.

CHAPTER 3

Teething is the Pits

*"But what am I? An infant crying in the night, an infant crying for the
light and with no language but a cry."*
A.L. Tennyson 1850

Imagine an 11-month old infant who has had very little
discomfort all his/her life suddenly experiencing very sensitive
gum tissue being ripped open by a sharp, erupting tooth. The
picture I've painted is my personal conception of how terrible
teething can be. On the other hand, some children pass through
this stage unaware that they should be crying and cranky day
and night. As a matter of fact, many pediatricians and pedodon-
tists believe that the child experiences no negative sensations
from teething. They say that "teething pain" is only mother's
catch-all excuse for the baby's crying behavior. If your child cries
when teething, these home remedies will help.

Buy over the counter numbing agents.

They work well for short periods of time to desensitize the gum
tissue. The act of placing the numbing agent on the teeth is
comforting to the child. Also, by rubbing the gums you are
removing bacteria that might be irritating the surrounding area
of the erupting tooth.

Feed the child food that is chewy such as toast, or bread sticks.

This stimulates the tissue
over the erupting tooth and
hastens the eruption time. Be
very careful that the child does
not choke on any foods that
he/she is given.

Plastic water-filled teething rings are often of value to
ease the pain of teething and
can be obtained in any pharmacy or child store. Keeping
the teething rings in the re-
frigerator before they are used
helps cool down the child's
inflamed gum tissue.

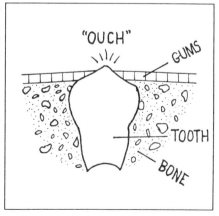

**Figure 5 - When a tooth erupts,
discomfort is possible.**

Some children may be irritable, have a low grade temperature, or diarrhea associated with teething.

Children's acetaminaphen (Tylenol), can often relieve the child's discomfort. Be sympathetic while your child is teething and give a little extra love and attention if it is required at this time. This stage will pass and you will not have spoiled your child.

Teeth may erupt with stains or other imperfections. This does not mean that other baby teeth or the permanent teeth will be imperfect.

The teeth may erupt crooked. About one month after erupting, the tongue and lips will usually move the teeth into the proper position.

Primary (baby) teeth will usually have spaces between them.

These spaces allow room for the larger, permanent teeth to erupt later in life. If there is a crowding problem in the baby set of teeth, there will usually be a problem of crowding with the permanent teeth. Early orthodontic guidance may be recommended for these children.

The child's dentition (teeth) will usually resemble one of the parent's. This will often give the parents and the dentist insight into the child's dental developmental pattern.

CHAPTER 4

Psychology of Avoiding Oral Fears

"The mind is a blank tablet upon which experience writes."
Rousseau

Children are very impressionable. If they see love, they will love. If they see happiness, they will be happy. If they see dental health care, they will practice dental health care.

It's our obligation to our children to demonstrate positive health habits that they can imitate. This imitation begins as soon as the child opens their eyes. Impressions are made from day one and these impressions are the foundations for the growing child.

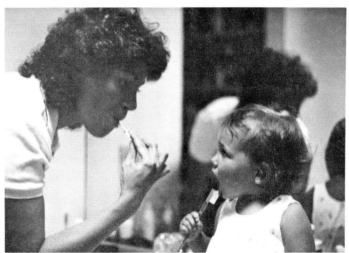

Figure 7

Practice good dental health care in front of your child. Rinse, brush and floss while your child is watching.

Show them that dental home care is an enjoyable experience.

Allow the child to have their own toothbrush. The soft bristles and plastic handle will not harm the developing teeth and gums. In fact, they will help clean them.

You must brush your children's teeth until they are at least five years old.

You can allow them to brush themselves, but you should

finalize their brushing episode by brushing their teeth for them. The teeth should be brushed at least twice a day, morning and evening.

Make this brushing experience enjoyable. Play a game while you are brushing your child's teeth. Make believe you are cleaning out some nasty villain such as Murky Dismal, Skeletor, or Lex Luthor as you brush away the plaque.

It is not necessary to use toothpaste for infants.

Wipe the child's developing teeth with a gauze pad or a soft toothbrush.

Your family should have a nutritionally balanced diet.

Supplement your child's diet with vitamins and minerals if necessary. This is helpful for the child's total development as well as for his/her dental health.

Feed your child chewy foods such as bread and apples. This stimulates growth of the oral complex (bone teeth and jaws) in a positive manner.

Be gentle when you approach your child's mouth with gauze or brush or liquid vitamins.

Do this with the child's approval. This is the beginning of creating a good or bad dental patient.

If you have had bad dental experiences, don't discuss them with, or impress them upon your children. Discuss them with your dentist.

If you are a good dental patient, bring your child with you to the dentist when you go in for your dental cleaning.

Allow your toddler to play in the dentist's waiting room while your spouse or other children receive dental treatment. This will help acquaint the toddler to the dental office.

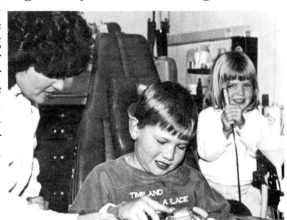

Figure 8

CHAPTER 5

The Basics of Home Dental Care

*You don't have to brush all your teeth,
only the ones you want to keep.*

Consider rinsing, brushing and flossing as a financial invest-ment as well as dental insurance. With proper home care you will decrease your dental bills considerably. Decay and periodontal disease will be less likely to occur, and dental repair will be minimal. The dental insurance you will receive will be derived from the old adage, "An ounce of prevention is worth a pound of cure".

You can keep your teeth forever!

By understanding the destructive process and using simple, inexpensive methods to avoid this destruction, you can maintain your dentition forever. Unfortunately, some people are lazy. They are too rushed in the morning and too tired in the evening to brush and floss. If you can find five minutes each day to dedicate to your oral hygiene, you will be investing in your overall health and insuring your longevity and the longevity of your teeth.

It is important to brush your teeth at least twice each day.

Brushing after each meal and snack is also recommended. Flossing once each day is suggested for proper oral health maintenance. The minimum oral health care routine should in-clude rinsing and brushing in the morning, and rinsing, brush-ing and flossing before bedtime. Children should follow the same routine.

However, instead of flossing, they can rinse with a fluoride solution at bedtime.

Food + Bacteria = Plaque

Plaque + Teeth + Gums = Destruction

Rinsing

- *Rinse with a pre–brushing dental rinse like Plax for 30 seconds to remove some plaque.* This will also loosen the remaining plaque which will make tooth brushing more effective.

Brushing

- *Use a soft or medium brush with rounded bristle ends.* When the brush is frayed or worn, get a new one. A toothbrush will usually last for four to six months. If the bristles become bent and frayed sooner, you are brushing too hard.
- *Aim the bristles of the brush toward the gum line at a 45° angle.* Use an organized approach to make sure you do not miss any tooth surfaces, (cheekside, tongueside, and biting surface). Use firm but gentle pressure and massage the gums and teeth in a circular fashion. Excessive brushing pressure may abrade and damage the tooth. (Handicapped children may have difficulty performing this necessary task. Ask your dentist about some tooth-brushing devices that are available to assist these special children.)

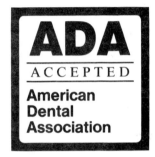

Figure 9

- *Use a toothpaste that has the ADA (American Dental Association) seal of approval.* Some of the newer anti-plaque toothpastes are also very good. Baking soda can also be an effective cleansing agent.

Flossing

Flossing enables you to clean areas that are inaccessible to the toothbrush:

- Wrap the floss (about 12 inches) around the middle fingers on each hand.
- Leave about 3 inches of unwrapped floss between your hands. Guide the floss gently between two teeth using your thumb and index fingers.
- Make sure that the floss goes slightly below the gum line.
- Move it up and down along the sides of each tooth.
- Begin by flossing the front teeth.

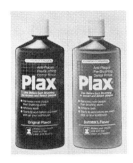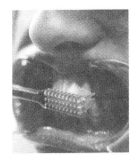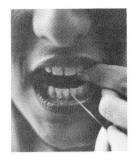

Figure 10 - Proper dental homecare includes rinsing, brushing and flossing.

- Floss the back teeth after you feel able and confident flossing the front teeth.
- Use waxed floss if you have difficulty getting the unwaxed floss between your teeth.

The floss should not get caught or fray on any fillings. If it does, inform your dentist of the problem area. If a filling is loosened by flossing, it is time for replacement. See your dentist.

You should floss between your child's molar teeth if possible.

Fluoride

Fluoride is a mineral that can become part of the tooth surface and internal structure. The tooth that has had the benefit of fluoride protection is considerably stronger and more resistant to decay than teeth that have not been treated with fluoride.

Fluoride treatment can be systemic or topical:

- **Systemic** - Systemic fluoride applications include fluoridated water or fluoride vitamins. This type of fluoride administration enables the developing tooth to incorporate fluoride into its total structure.
- **Topical** - Topical fluoride treatments include fluoride rinses, fluoride toothpaste, and professional dental fluoride applications. This technique provides a protective fluoride coat on the surface layer of the tooth.

Periodic fluoride application by your dentist is highly recommended.

Fluoride rinses at home are very helpful and also highly recommended.

If your child is not a routine fluoride rinser, there are special fluoride rinses your dentist can prescribe that can be used once a week instead of on a daily basis. If you are not drinking fluoridated water, you should ask your dentist to prescribe a fluoride vitamin supplement.

Children who are too young to "swish and spit" should not be allowed to use toothpaste in large quantities or swallow fluoride rinses. Excessive amounts of fluoride may stain the developing teeth (fluorosis).

Special fluoride applications from your dentist will often reduce or eliminate hypersensitivity (sensitive teeth). This will also help to prevent recurrent cavities. This fluoride procedure is mostly for adults.

Other dental devices

Additional dental cleaning devices DO NOT eliminate the need for brushing and flossing. When used in conjunction with other home care techniques they may surely help to maintain a healthy oral environment.

Water Pic, electric toothbrushes, toothpicks, stimudents, proxybrushes, floss holders, and floss threaders are some of the extra dental care devices you may want to consider using.

Disclosing Tablets

Disclosing tablets or disclosing drops can be purchased from your pharmacy or your dentist. These tablets contain a food coloring which will visually demonstrate where plaque is collecting around your teeth and gums.

Brushing and flossing after using a disclosing tablet will allow you to make sure that all of the plaque has been removed.

Visiting the dentist at least two to four times a year is reasonable and necessary. Dental visits can begin as early as age two.

If the dentist recommends more frequent cleaning visits, follow his/her advice.

There are four phases of dental treatment:
1. **Examination:** The teeth, soft tissues, occlusion (bite), and general health should be thoroughly evaluated prior to any major therapy.
2. **Reconstruction:** Removal of decay, elimination of periodontal disease, abscesses and cysts, and replacement of missing teeth.
3. **Maintenance:**. professional checkups (exams) and dental cleanings are necessary to maintain the reconstruction that has been performed.

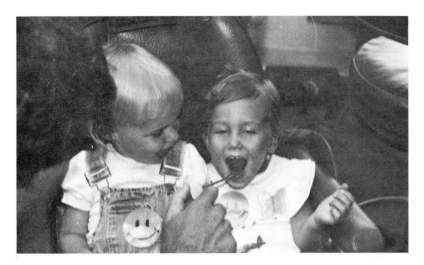

Figure 11 - Dental Visits can be fun.

4. Repair: Dental reconstruction does not last forever. Fillings, crowns and dentures must be replaced from time to time. The time between replacing dental work varies for each individual. Some of these variables that determine how long your dental work will last include; the dentist's ability, the patient's home care and diet, the materials used, the existing dental state prior to reconstruction and the professional maintenance of the reconstruction.

CHAPTER 6

The First Dental Visit

"A sound mind in a sound body is a short but full description of a happy state in this world."
John Locke 1693

By the time your child is three years old, he/she should have had his/her first visit to the dentist. This can be as little as a ride in the dental chair and counting of the teeth, or as extensive as a cleaning, exam, fluoride treatment, and tooth-brushing instructions. Your child's receptiveness will determine how much the dentist or hygienist will do.

A child's behavior in the dental office is mostly determined by his/her parents, siblings and peers.

Children will usually go to the dentist with a preconceived notion of what will happen to them. If they have been negatively prepared, the visit may be a failure. If they have been properly prepared, the experience will be enjoyable.

Early cavity detection and treatment is essential for proper patient and dental management.

Help your child's attitude toward dentistry to be a positive one.

Discuss with them the good experiences you have had at your dental visits.

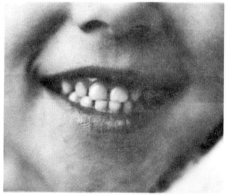
Figure 12 - At age three all of the baby teeth are present.

Choose your child's dentist wisely (see Chapter 24).

Make the first dental visit in the morning. Children are usually more open minded early in the day. By the afternoon, children are often tired and easily upset.

Do not allow your child to have any high sugar concentration food (candy) before the dental visit. Sugar in the child's system has a tendency to make them hyperactive. This behavior is not conducive to a relaxed dental visit.

If you communicate well with your child at this age you can

inform him/her on the day of the appointment what he or she might expect in general terms.

If the child is anxious (nervous), sometimes minimal parental forewarning is better. The dentist and staff are trained to inform the first-timer of what to expect.

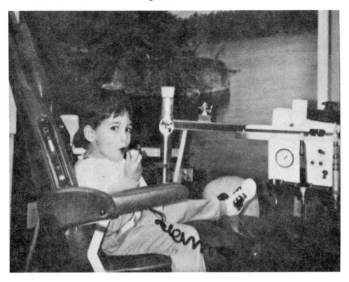

Figure 13 -

If the child is willing to be with the hygienist or dentist without Mom or Dad, let them.

You are not needed. The hygienist or dentist should discuss their findings with you after the appointment. If you are concerned about a specific dental problem, tell the hygienist, dentist, or receptionist before the child is examined.

It is good for the child to establish his or her own rapport with the dentist. This will be a long term friendship that can begin with the first encounter.

If the child needs your presence, go with them to the treatment room. Do not stand right by the chair holding their hand and waiting to comfort them. This will not help the situation, only hinder it.

Let the dentist or hygienist do the talking.

Do not interrupt their line of discussion. You will only distract your child and make the situation more difficult for the professional.

If possible, walk out of the room several times to sever the parental dependence slowly. If the child appears comfortable, ask him/her if you may leave for a few minutes to talk with the receptionist.

Be sure to advise the receptionist and dentist about any important medical conditions your child might have before any treatment is performed.

Allergies, heart conditions requiring pre-medication, and bleeding problems are some of the conditions your dentist should be informed about.

Inform the dentist of any possible speech problems your child might have. Tongue thrusting, tongue tied, and malocclusions can add to your child's speech problem. Your dentist and a speech therapist can often help the child overcome a speech problem before any serious ramifications occur.

At the end of the visit thank the dentist or hygienist, co-ordinate future appointments with the receptionist, and leave the office with a *smile.*

CHAPTER 7

Reinforcing Good Dental Behavior

"Any subject can be taught effectively in some intellectually honest form to any child at any stage of development."
J.S. Bruner 1960

I do not advocate psyching your children up to have them perform properly: however it can, at times, be very effective. It is easier to verbally reward your child when he/she has had a good dental visit than to drag them by the ear to return to the dentist.

It is too often forgotten that a kind word is better than a handful of store bought rewards. Hug your children, pat them on the head, smile at them and tell them you are proud of them when you leave the dental office. If they behave well during the office visit, let them know it. After the dental experience, discuss with the child what happened.

Let the child tell you what the dentist did. It was their day, so let them relate their experience to you and others.

Be positive in your responses and reinforce the child's good feelings of how well he or she behaved.

At the dinner table repeat the positive experience to your spouse or other children. "Bobby rode in the chair, had his teeth counted, and the dentist even used the electric toothpolisher to clean his teeth. What a *big* boy he was!" The word big is very important to children. It connotes adulthood more than any other adjective.

If the child did not behave well at the office, allow your spouse or a friend to take him or her back for the next visit to the dentist.

Often, the child will behave better with another adult at the second visit.

If your child has had a bad experience, wait a few weeks and try again.

After several return visits, your child should be more receptive to the dental treatment.

If your child is adamant about not returning to the dentist or hygienist, do not force a return visit to the same dentist but consider visiting a specialist such as a pedodontist.

Do not over-react to a child's negative behavior.

Your over reaction to such behavior can only induce more fear associated with a dental visit. Inform the child of your love for them but state that you are dissatisfied with the unacceptable behavior.

Candy and other foods with abundant sugar content will lead to increased destruction of teeth unless moderation is used.

Brushing after eating candy is recommended. Never threaten a child with cavities for eating candy or poor brushing habits. These tactics make the dentist's job much more difficult.

Encourage fruits and vegetables as snacks. These foods are less destructive to the teeth, and are beneficial to the rest of the body.

CHAPTER 8

The First cavity

"The most prevalent noncontagious disease is a dental cavity."
Trivial Pursuit Card

Cavities are one of life's minor displeasures. They happen to most people even if they brush 500 times a day. If your child has a cavity, have it taken care of quickly. Cavities, when detected early, are quickly and painlessly treated. The use of an anesthetic (novocaine) is usually not necessary. Advanced cavities are also easily treated (anesthetics may be required).

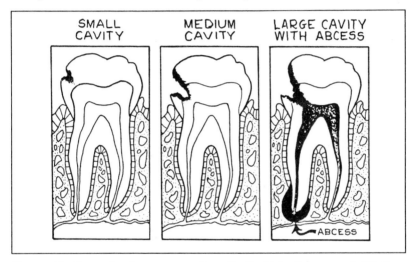

SMALL CAVITY   MEDIUM CAVITY   LARGE CAVITY WITH ABCESS

ABCESS

Figure 15 - Decay begins as a small cavity (hole) in the enamel. If left untreated, it will progress and finally form an abscess.

Do not upset your child with fearful words like drill, needle, fillings, or pain.

Here is a sample of how you might inform your child of his/her dental cavity visit:

Mom: Jamie, we are going to see that nice dentist again.

Son: What is he going to do?

Mom: He is going to clean one of your teeth a little better.

Son: Why?

Mom: There are some spots on the tooth that have to be cleaned before the spots get any bigger.

Son: What will he use?

Mom: He will probably use his electric toothbrush. He may also use a rounded tooth cleaner and water.

Son: Will I get a needle? (Some children have heard through the grapevine of the infamous needle.)

Mom: I don't think so. The dentist might want to put your tooth to sleep for a little while, but that's kind of easy.

Son: Is it going to hurt?

Mom: I don't believe so. If you open your mouth wide and let the dentist clean the tooth, we'll be finished quickly. Then we'll have a special day together.

Note: That is the truth. If your dentist is good (see Chapter 24) and your child behaves, most visits can be pleasant. Your discussion with your child will vary, but the general ideas I have outlined for you should help direct your responses to his/her questions.

1. Be honest.

2. Use words that do not sound painful or threatening.

3. Avoid words that their friends might have used if they have had negative dental experiences.

4. If you are not sure how to answer a question, let him or her ask the dentist.

Novocaine, a local anesthesia (the "needle"), may not be necessary. When cavities are detected early, decay removal can be accomplished easily without the need for anesthesia.

X-rays should be taken periodically

X-rays should be taken periodically (6 months to a year) for early detection of growth progress, cavity formation, deformities, and other possible problems.

Dental sealants are one way to avoid drilling and filling.

By placing a plastic coating on top of potential decay areas, cavities may be circumvented. Ask your dentist about this technique.

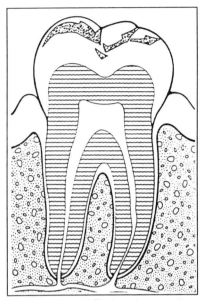 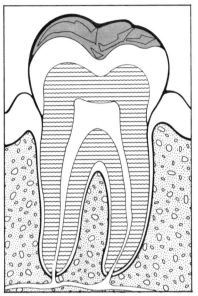

The permanent first molar erupts at age 6. This tooth can stay healthy forever. Grooves and contours of the tooth allow plaque to remain on the tooth surface for extended periods of time. This will lead to decay of this tooth.

A plastic coating (sealant) is placed on the surface of this tooth. This creates a smooth surface that prevents plaque accumulation. This will prevent the tooth from decaying.

Figure 16

Children with advanced dental problems.

Children with advanced dental problems (large cavities, abscesses, and/or behavioral problems may require pre-medication, nitrous oxide, or general anesthesia for dental treatment. There may be some discomfort involved with these major cases. It may be advisable to utilize a specialist's (pedodontist) expertise for these situations.

CHAPTER 9

The Tooth Fairy Cometh

"...and it fell out while I was eating a Twinkie."
Mathewson Third Grader

By the age of seven, your child is maturing rapidly. One of the most obvious changes during the early growth years happen when their first front permanent tooth begins to erupt. This usually happens between six and eight years of age. It is usually preceded by the loss of a baby tooth... this is often more traumatic for Mom and Dad than it is for the child. The suggestions in this Chapter will answer many common questions.

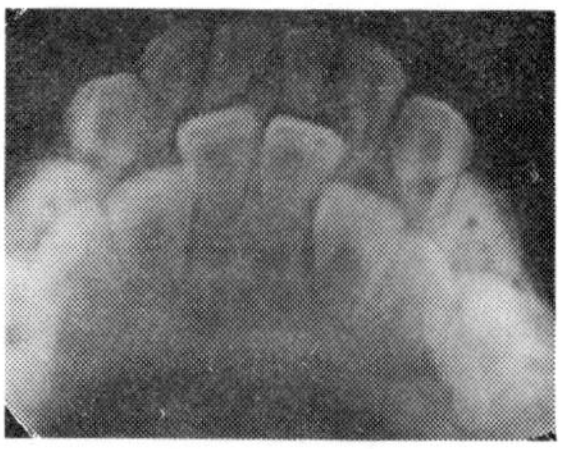

Figure 17 - This x-ray shows that the permanent teeth are developing underneath the baby teeth. These baby teeth will be lost soon.

There is often discomfort just prior to the loss of a tooth.

Every time the loose tooth moves, it irritates the gums and your child may be uncomfortable.

Tylenol, or another mild pain medication taken orally for one or two days will lessen the child's discomfort and will usually enable him or her to loosen the tooth without parental help. **Never** place aspirin on a tooth or irritated gum tissue. You will cause a severe aspirin burn of the cheek and gum tissue.

The dentist may have to remove the baby tooth if the child is unable to loosen it. This is usually an easy and painless procedure.

Frequently, the permanent tooth will partially erupt before the baby tooth is lost.

If this condition persists for more than two months, consult your dentist. Your child may need professional help to remove the loose baby tooth.

To help your child lose his or her baby teeth, try these home remedies when the tooth is very loose.

1. Feed him/her corn on the cob with dinner.
2. Feed him/her apples for snacking.
3. Let him/her chew sugarless gum.

The idea behind these tricks is that while eating these foods, the child will apply enough pressure on the loose tooth to facilitate its departure,

If the tooth is hanging by a thread with just a bit of gum tissue holding it in, and your child is afraid to finish what he/she began, place an ice cube on the area and let your child hold it for about 10 or 20 minutes.

When the area is desensitized, a gentle fingerhold on the tooth followed be a quick twist and pull motion will remove the tooth.

Allowing your child to rinse with ice water followed by vigorous tooth brushing may also facilitate the loss of the tooth.

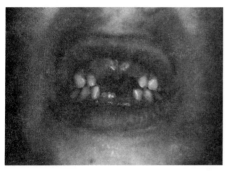

Figure 18 - Permanent teeth do not always erupt immediately after the baby teeth are lost.

Your child should be checked by the dentist on a regular basis to be certain of proper development.

X-rays may be necessary to check on the tooth loss and eruption process.

Mixed dentition (permanent and baby teeth), might look unpleasant. The two permanent central teeth will often erupt with a space between them.

This space usually closes as the other permanent teeth erupt. They may also look crowded and misaligned. This often straightens without the dentist's help. Any major development problems can always be corrected orthodontically.

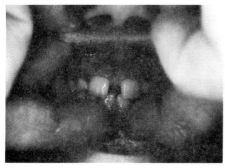

Figure 19 - These two permanent central teeth will move together and the space will disappear in the next six months.

The six-year molars (first molars), are often the first permanent teeth to erupt.

It is usually very difficult for the child to properly brush these permanent molars. Because of this, these teeth usually become decayed. Make it your responsibility to check and brush these important permanent molars. Sealants are highly recommended for these permanent molars.

CHAPTER 10

Dental Injuries

"If anything can go wrong, it will, usually at the worst possible time."
Murphy's Law #1

"Boys will be boys," Jeff's Mom said as Jeff sat in the dental chair. Jeff had fractured his brand new permanent central incisor tooth. Her trust in her dentist and the knowledge that Jeff's tooth could be repaired made this situation less traumatic than it could have been.

Bicycles, swimming pools, and stairs are notorious for chipping and fracturing front teeth. Children of all ages are susceptible to accidents.

If a child falls and fractures a tooth, do not panic. Your reaction to the situation cues your child as to how many tears need be shed. If Mom gets excited, the child believes he or she must be seriously hurt, then tears and fears take over.

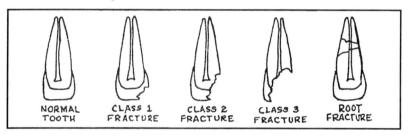

NORMAL TOOTH   CLASS 1 FRACTURE   CLASS 2 FRACTURE   CLASS 3 FRACTURE   ROOT FRACTURE

Figure 20 - Possible treatments:

Class 1 Fracture
- Smooth the tooth
- Fluoride treatment
- Office bonding

Class 2 Fracture
- Pin buildup
- Veneer bonding
- Crown

Class 3 Fracture
- Bonding
- Root canal
- Post and crown

Root Fracture
- Root canal
- Bonding stabilization
- Post stabilization
- Extraction and implant reconstruction

In the event of a traumatic tooth injury, assess the situation and react accordingly.

1. Examine the child for any other injuries.
2. Clean dirt and blood off the facial, mouth, area.
3. Re-evaluate the damage.
4. Place ice on the lip area.
5. Do not put ice on or near the tooth.
6. For Class 2 and 3 fractures (see chart) see the

dentist as soon as possible that day. For Class 1 fractures see the dentist soon.

7. For completely knocked out teeth, see the dentist immediately.

Often a fall will cause front baby teeth to be lost prematurely. This is not uncommon and is usually no cause for alarm. Visits to the dentist are not always necessary when this happens.

If a permanent tooth is completely knocked out:

1. Keep calm and place ice on the lip area.
2. Find the tooth and gently clean it.
3. Wrap it in a moist paper towel, cloth, or in a glass of milk.
4. See your dentist immediately with your child and the tooth. The greatest success for re-implantation occurs within one hour of the accident.
5. If your dentist is unavailable, call an oral surgeon, another dentist or go to a hospital.
6. The dentist may be able to re-position the avulsed (knocked-out) tooth and bond it in place. This re-implantation can last for several years, or possibly forever.
7. Root canal therapy might be necessary to remove the injured pulp tissue at a later date.
8. If the re-implantation does not work, there are several ways to replace the lost tooth. These will be discussed in a later Chapter.

Accidents may cause muscle spasms of the jaw.

Muscle relaxant medication from your dentist or physician can effectively relieve the discomfort. Warm, moist compresses will also help to alleviate the pain.

Injured teeth will often turn dark.

This indicates internal tooth damage. An X-ray should be taken and your dentist should decide what the recommended course of action should be.

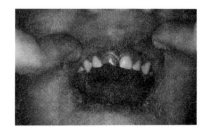

Figure 21 - This baby tooth was traumatized, turned dark, and is in need of treatment.

Possible treatments for traumatized *baby* teeth.

1. Examine the tooth monthly and make sure no further damage results to it, or to the developing permanent tooth.

2. Repair the tooth with bonding techniques or capping if needed.

3. Remove the injured tooth in order to prevent injury to the developing permanent tooth.

4. Perform root canal therapy to save the baby tooth for space and aesthetic maintenance.

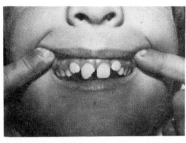 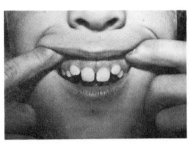

Figure 22 - This permanent tooth was damaged accidently (dental fracture)

The damaged tooth was repaired in the dental office with a bonding procedure.

Prevention of accidents is the best solution to avoiding dental injuries.

Child-proof your house. Areas which are potentially dangerous should be safeguarded:

1. Put rubber corners on coffee tables.

2. Tack down loose, movable throw rugs.

3. Explain the dangers of running down stairs to your child.

4. You and your child must wear seat belts when riding in a car. (It's the law). Dental injuries are routinely associated with car accidents.

5. Warn your child against reckless bike riding and skateboarding.

6. If your child plays sports, be sure that he/she wears a mouthguard.

Types of mouthguards:
Sold in sporting goods stores:

1. Pre made: Small, medium, or large.

2. Heat treated. First placed in hot water. It will adapt to fit the teeth accurately.

Custom made:

3. Made by the dentist for a custom fit. The 'Rolls Royce' of mouth guards.

CHAPTER 11

The Orthodontics Story

When you're smiling, the whole world smiles with you.

Orthodontic treatment for you or your child is one of the best investments you can make. Consider the money that you spend over a lifetime improving your house, car, or boat. These objects consume thousands of dollars and return only temporary pleasure. Your teeth on the other hand, are used throughout your entire life and provide you with both physical and aesthetic health benefits. Orthodontics can be considered as the fine tuning of your teeth. Just as a car engine runs better and lasts longer when tuned properly, so does your tooth complex. In the long run, the expense of braces is a wise investment.

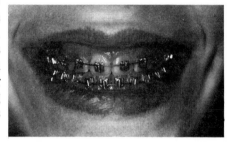

Figure 23 The classic orthodontic smile

Orthodontic treatment

Orthodontic treatment will properly align the front and back teeth and jaws to achieve the maximum chewing efficiency of your particular system. Proper chewing is needed to diminish food size, which aids digestion and improves your total health. Orthodontic treatment will also eliminate crowed teeth which is a major cause of decay and gum disease.

There are 20 baby teeth (10 upper, 10 lower). At about age 7 the baby teeth begin to be replaced by permanent teeth. There will be 32 (16 upper, 16 lower) permanent teeth. Normal growth and development will create enough room for these additional 12 teeth. Sometimes, however, there is a need for orthodontic assistance to direct this growth properly.

Orthodontic treatment for adults is very common.

It not only improves the alignment and function of the teeth, but it usually makes individuals feel much better about themselves. It adds to confidence and improves their general outlook on life.

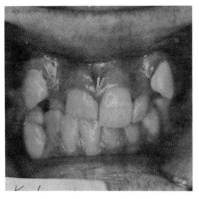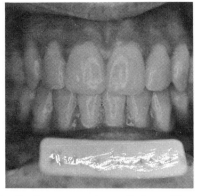

Figure 24 - After two years of orthodontic therapy, a dramatic transition can be seen.

Functional orthodontic appliances

Functional orthodontic appliances between the ages of 8 and 12 can often improve the total orthodontic picture. Treatment is often easier and extractions might not be necessary. Consult your dentist or orthodontist.

Orthodontic treatment is easier than you think.

With modern orthodontic bonding techniques, treatment usually takes one to three years, depending on the type of treatment involved. The cost will vary for your particular treatment, depending on the specific problem. payments can usually be spread over a period of time, which helps to make this worthwhile investment financially easier to manage.

In certain cases surgical re-positioning of the upper or lower jaw may be necessary to allow orthodontic therapy to obtain maximum results. The surgery involved is often quick and relatively painless.

Bonding brackets to the teeth is a newer and easier technique for the patient and dentist.

Consult your dentist or orthodontist if bonding, as opposed to banding can be used for treatment.

Invisible braces is a new technique which can only be done with certain cases. This technique involves the bonding of orthodontic brackets on the inside portion of the teeth, as opposed to the outside or visible part of the teeth.

Parafunctional habits

Parafunctional habits (thumb-sucking, cheek-biting, lip-sucking) are a major cause of misaligned teeth. Early detection and elimination of these habits can prevent orthodontic problems.

Early diagnosis and treatment of orthodontic problems usually make the case easier to treat and decreases the amount of time necessary for completion of the case.

Once braces are in place, extra care is necessary to prevent decay and gum disease.

Plaque easily builds up around the wires and must be removed with proper brushing at least three times a day. Frequent professional cleanings two to four times a year are advisable.

Rinsing with a pre–rinse before brushing is great for people with braces and other orthodontic appliances because the rinse can reach anywhere in the mouth. It works to help remove plaque even in places where it's difficult to brush.

Avoid foods that might snap the wires or chip off the brackets (i.e. gum, nuts, frozen candy bars, or any hard food item).

Make sure to rinse with a fluoride solution daily.

The use of a water pic on a low setting is highly recommended during orthodontic treatment.

CHAPTER 12

Teenage Dental Care

"Bid them wash their faces and keep their teeth clean."
Shakespeare - 1606

"She never listens to me." "I tell him to brush his teeth or he'll lose them all." "She's too busy watching TV." Parents repeat phrases such as these to dentists all over the world when told how many cavities their teenager has. This Chapter is intended to give parents the upper hand when dealing with a teenager's dental neglect.

These are cavity prone years.

It is not uncommon to find cavities in the mouths of even the best dental care kids. Early detection and treatment of these cavities can save the child discomfort at a later date.

During puberty, your child's hormones are very active. Hormonal changes and poor dental hygiene habits can lead to bleeding gums and bad breath. A professional cleaning and improved dental home care, rinsing, brushing and flossing, at least twice a day will help to eliminate this problem.

Make sure that your teenager visits the dentist twice a year for dental cleanings and examinations.

Professional exams decrease the chances of undiagnosed cavities and gum disease.

If your teenager goes to sleep without brushing, place a toothbrush on their pillow as a subtle hint.

If they don't brush in the morning, place the toothbrush on the breakfast plate.

If their toothbrush is worn out, get them a new one.

Cut out pictures of people with ugly teeth and leave them around their rooms.

Repeated nagging is counterproductive while humorous hints are more effective.

Keep the number of snacks per day to a minimum.

Impress upon the teenager that decay producing acids form each time a snack is eaten.

Ask your dentist for disclosing tablets. This red stain will vividly show remaining plaque on your child's teeth. This may 'gross' them out' enough to motivate an improvement in home dental care techniques.

Be aware of your child's nutritional needs.

The developing teenager needs the proper vitamins, minerals, and nutrients to help build strong bones and body tissues. (See Chapter 21).

If your child is involved in a contact sport:

Be sure that a mouthguard is used. Refer to Chapter 10 for an overview of mouthguard differences.

The chewing surfaces of the molars (back teeth) are the most susceptible to decay.

Extra care should be taken to brush these teeth well. Many dentists are using sealants on molars as extra protection. A thin layer of clear plastic is bonded to the biting surface and can last anywhere from two to ten years, protecting teeth from decay. When a sealant wears off, it can easily be replaced by the dentist if necessary.

CHAPTER 13

The Wisdom about Wisdom Teeth

Wisdom teeth are time bombs waiting to explode.

What are they?

Wisdom teeth are the third molar teeth.

Where are they located?

They can be found in the upper and lower jaws in the back of the mouth. These teeth are usually the last teeth to erupt.

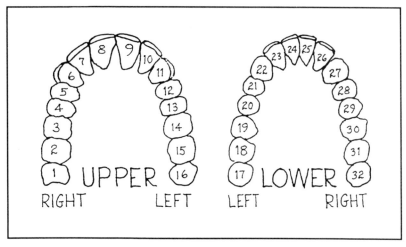

Figure 25A - Numbers 1, 16, 17 and 32 are the wisdom teeth.

Why are they?

Throughout human evolution, there has been a constant change in the size of the head and jaws. With the passage of time, the human head has become smaller, and the size of the jaw has also decreased. Once, the wisdom teeth were a necessary part of the chewing apparatus; presently, they serve little or no purpose.

When are they?

They usually erupt between 18 to 20 years of age. Often they can remain impacted (not erupted) forever.

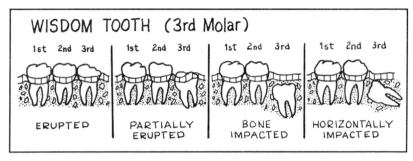

WISDOM TOOTH (3rd Molar)

| 1st 2nd 3rd | 1st 2nd 3rd | 1st 2nd 3rd | 1st 2nd 3rd |
| ERUPTED | PARTIALLY ERUPTED | BONE IMPACTED | HORIZONTALLY IMPACTED |

Figure 25B - Different stages of wisdom tooth eruption.

Who cares?

You do! Wisdom teeth will usually be a cause of dental discomfort sooner or later. This discomfort (often extremely painful) can be avoided.

How do I avoid wisdom tooth discomfort?

Discuss with your dentist your particular dental architecture to determine what course of treatment should be taken. He/she may recommend that you have them removed. Ask to see the X-rays of these teeth so you can see what he/she is talking about.

What problems can wisdom teeth cause?

The wisdom tooth can decay and lead to an abscess, which can cause severe pain. (According to Murphy's Law, this pain will usually occur at the most inopportune time.)

The gum tissue around the wisdom tooth and the neighboring second molar (an important tooth), may become sore and infected. The wisdom tooth may create a food trap, causing food to collect and decay the second molar's root. This may be impossible to restore.

Due to its position in the dental arch, TMJ pain and dysfunction are often caused by misaligned wisdom teeth. The TMJ (Temperomandibular joint) will be discussed in Chapter 23.

Impacted wisdom teeth have the potential for abscess and cyst formation (time bombs in the dental arch).

As you age, removal of the wisdom teeth can become more and more difficult. Recovery from wisdom tooth extraction is usually uneventful for the young adult.

In certain cases, a wisdom tooth can be utilized in restoring a debilitated area. If a teenager must lose a permanent first molar, it may be possible to remove and re-implant the third molar (wisdom tooth) into this first molar position.

Basic Wisdom Rules

Keep them:

> If there is enough room for them.
>
> If they are easily brushed and flossed.
>
> If they function properly for chewing.
>
> If they are not decayed.
>
> If they are not periodontally compromised.
>
> If they are necessary to rebuild areas where teeth are missing.
>
> If they do not interfere with the occlusion (bite).
>
> If they do not irritate the cheeks while chewing.

Remove them:

> If your dentist recommends that you have them removed.
>
> If you doubt the wisdom of his or her recommendation, get a second opinion.
>
> If your wisdom teeth do not fulfill *all* of the preceding requirements, you are probably better off without them.

CHAPTER 14

College Years: "I'll Brush My Teeth Tomorrow"

"Wake up Bob! The party is over. Go brush your teeth."
A.B. 1972

Your children are no longer children: they are young adults. Their dental habits should be well established.

Your young adults should now take responsibility to maintain their dental health by arranging dental visits during their college breaks, at least twice a year. They should make appointments with their dentist several weeks, or months ahead; these vacation times are usually very busy times for your dentist. Finding a last minute appointment before the student returns to school might be difficult.

Treat the student as an adult.

Appeal to their intellect to motivate their dental home care without nagging.

Most of their reconstructive work (fillings) was probably completed before entering college. If so, maintenance should be the only dental treatment necessary at this time.

When you send a "care package", include a toothbrush and some toothpaste. Toiletries are low on the priority list of the college student.

Occasionally ask the student how his or her teeth are doing.

You might be surprised if he/she tells you he/she has a problem. He/she might not tell you if you don't ask.

College students usually find third molars (wisdom teeth) erupting about this time and can be very uncomfortable.

Here are some wisdom remedies to calm painful tooth eruption:

1. Be sure to rinse and brush the gum tissue overlying the erupting tooth. This may be uncomfortable at first, but it will help to cleanse the area and ease the discomfort.
2. Rinse with warm salt water. (8 oz. water to 1 tsp.

salt.) Often, this will ease the discomfort.

3. Analgesics such as Tylenol will also ease the discomfort.
4. See a dentist if the discomfort persists.
5. Have the third molars removed if your dentist recommends this.

Simple painless cleaning of the area will solve the problem temporarily. An antibiotic might also be necessary.

School pre-exam time is notorious for gingivitis, commonly called bleeding gums or trenchmouth.

The added exam time stress and dental neglect are contributing factors to these problems. These conditions will usually heal with proper care (rinsing, brushing and flossing and professional cleaning).

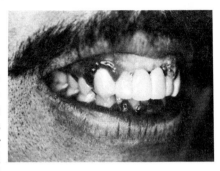

Figure 26 - This gum tissue is very tender and in need of immediate attention

Solutions to gingivitis:

1. Brush the affected gum tissue frequently. It will bleed considerably, but this will help to shorten the duration of the problem.
2. Massage gums with the index finger to stimulate blood circulation and promote healing.
3. Floss. Make sure that the floss goes slightly below the gumline for adequate plaque removal.
4. Rinse with warm salt water.
5. See the dentist or hygienist for a professional cleaning.
6. College health offices can usually refer the out of town student to a local dentist if necessary.
7. Early detection and treatment of this serious dental problem is necessary to avoid a full scale infection.
8. Novelty college habits such as chewing tobacco, snuff, pipe smoking, cigars, etc. should be discouraged. These habits may cause severe dental problems. Oral and systemic cancer are other potential dangers associated with these habits.

CHAPTER 15

The Critical Years ... 25 to 40

"The most perishable commodity is time. It is here and then it's gone, never to be seen again."
C. S. 1980

"I'm working full time. I have a family to take care of. I don't have time to go to the dentist." Nonsense. If you had a toothache you would find the time and money necessary to visit a dentist. Because your parents are no longer setting up your 6 month cleaning and exam appointments does not mean that your teeth have a clean bill of health for the rest of your life. As a maturing adult, you must now assume the responsibility of maintaining your own oral health and health in general.

You can keep your teeth forever, easily, inexpensively, and without discomfort.

It is much less expensive to maintain good oral health than it is to repair and rebuild what has been destroyed. If repair and reconstruction have been performed, maintenance is of the utmost importance. If major dental treatment is maintained properly, it will last much longer than if it were neglected. Fillings do not last forever. Replacement of old worn fillings is often necessary to prevent recurrent decay and tooth fractures.

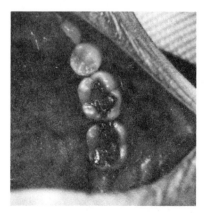

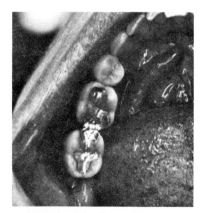

Figure 27 - These old fillings need to be replaced. Broken and worn margins have allowed decay to form under these fillings.

Figure 28 - New replacement fillings are properly contoured, have clean margins, and the decay has been removed.

At this stage in your life, gum disease (periodontal disease or pyorrhea) is the major destroyer of the masticatory system.

The gum tissue must be properly maintained in order to support the teeth for the rest of your life.

Some signs of gum disease include:
- Bad breath
- Loose teeth
- Bleeding gums
- Irregular gum tissue contour
- Puss draining from the gums
- Pain when the gums or tooth are touched
- Swollen gums

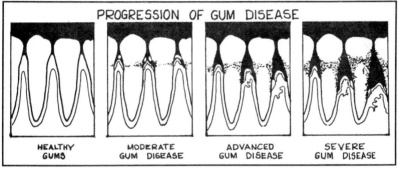

Figure 28A - Early detection and treatment of gum disease is highly recommended.

Gum disease can often be detected by the dentist.

He/she might measure the pocket depth around each tooth. The pocket depth is the distance between the height of the gum tissue and the height of the bone. The deeper the pocket, the greater the bone loss. The greater the bone loss, the greater the chances of losing the tooth.

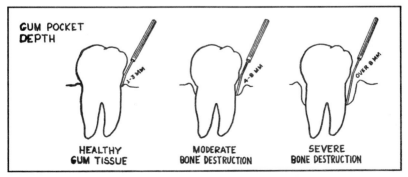

Figure 28B - Dental probes can measure the pocket depth.

Pocket depth measurements should be taken periodically, one to four times a year.

Remember, early detection of a problem results in easier and less expensive treatment to remedy that problem.

The tooth and bone support are in a 3-dimensional world. It is possible to have bone destruction on one side of the tooth and healthy bone on all the other sides.

Rinse with Plax before brushing. This will help to loosen the plaque from the surface of the teeth. Brushing and flossing will now be more effective.

Its pleasant taste and ease of use makes it easy to include in your daily oral regimen.

Flossing may be time consuming, but it is a necessary part of proper dental home care.

Flossing may save you from needing periodontal therapy in the future.

Dry brushing can lessen and possibly eliminate gum disease.

While you perform a mindless task (e.g., watching TV) you can take a brush and massage the gum tissue. The fluid (and possibly blood) that accumulates can be spit into a paper cup. If this is done during an entire program (1/2 to 1 hour each day) the physical stimulation will activate the gum tissue, remove plaque and eventually decrease the harmful effects of gum disease. Be sure that you follow the correct brushing techniques outlined in Chapter 5. Excessive scrubbing may damage the tooth... however, correct gum stimulation will be beneficial.

Additional home care aids.

Additional home care aids include stimudents, water pics, electric toothbrushes, rubber-tip gum massagers, etc. These are also helpful for dental health maintenance.

If a filling is lost during flossing, the filling was in need of replacement.

Don't blame the floss for loosening a filling; thank it for finding a defective restoration.

If your gums are not healthy, more frequent cleanings might be necessary. Ask your dentist if your gums need a professional cleaning more often (3 or 4 times a year).

If your gums have receded

If your gums have receded, the exposed part of the tooth may be sensitive to touch or hot and cold liquids. This gumline sensitivity can often be alleviated with some simple techniques.

Special desensitizing toothpastes, used daily, will coat the tooth with a fluoride barrier and decrease its sensitivity.

The Dentist can electrically desensitize the gumline area of the tooth with a special dental device. Or, he/she can place a plastic coating over the sensitive tooth area which will further alleviate the discomfort.

The use of baking soda, peroxide, and salt may help the gum tissue look better but in fact does not cure gum disease. Do not be misled by this surface application. Consult your dentist or periodontist before using this technique.

It is also possible for gums to recede because of improper brushing. Consult your dentist if your gums are receding.

T.M.J. (Temporomandibular Joint)

The occlusion (the way the teeth come together) must work harmoniously with the T.M.J. If it does not, there will be a constant muscle and joint irritation which might reflect itself with painful symptoms and eventual destruction of the teeth, gums, bone, and joint. Headaches, neck aches, backaches, clicking jaw, facial and muscle spasms, are some symptoms of a T.M.J. problem. TMJ disorders and remedies are discussed in Chapter 23.

CHAPTER 16

It's Never Too Late To Get Your Dental House In Order

"Never say never"
J. Z. 1986

Congratulations. You have made it through the difficult oral care years and you have all of your own teeth functioning to 100% efficiency. You enjoy your meals, chewing is not a problem, digestion is normal, and you look 20 years younger than your friends who have not cared for their teeth. All you have to do now is continue rinsing, brushing and flossing and visiting your dentist several times a year for professional cleanings.

Unfortunately, most middle-aged people continue to have dental problems. Your teeth are even more uncomfortable now, and you've got to do something about it. It may be a single tooth that has been a problem all along. It may be a gum problem which has allowed the teeth to loosen up to a level of major discomfort and embarrassment. It might be that you are totally fed up with your teeth and want a dental solution once and for all.

If you are nodding your head, this Chapter is for you. The children are grown, the bills are manageable, and your life is in order. But you may not enjoy chewing properly. You owe yourself some good and complete dental treatment.

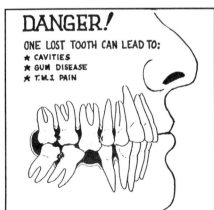

DANGER!

ONE LOST TOOTH CAN LEAD TO:
★ CAVITIES
★ GUM DISEASE
★ T.M.J. PAIN

Figure 29 - The loss of one tooth can lead to major destruction in the future.

If you haven't been to the dentist in a very long time, put away your fears and listen to what he/she has to say about your particular situation.

Inform him or her of any change in your medical history such as new medications, allergies, heart problems, etc.

New fillings might be sensitive to cold temperatures.

This sensation fades in time. New fillings might also feel and taste metallic. The sensation should decrease in one or two days. If it doesn't disappear, have your dentist adjust the filling.

If you have periodontal disease, proper therapy might enable the dentist to save several, if not all of your teeth for the rest of your life.

If he/she can save only a few teeth, these can be used to support replacement teeth such as an overdenture or bridge work.

Dental restoration is architectural reconstruction on a small scale. It is an attempt to duplicate as much as possible the original oral structure. To support false teeth, you need a good foundation. This includes the gums, bone, and remaining teeth. Your dentist can recommend several possible treatment plans, and your involvement will help you understand and make the treatment that much more rewarding and enjoyable.

Take good care of your new oral reconstruction.

The new crowns, bridges or partial dentures that have been made need special care. Impeccable home care of rinsing, brushing and flossing, along with routine professional cleanings are imperative to maintain what has been reconstructed.

Your new dental work should feel comfortable, smooth, and look natural.

If the work that has been performed does not feel good, tell the dentist. Do not ignore the problem, it might get worse.

New dentures, partial and full, might have sore spots which cause pain or ulcerations. See the dentist to adjust the denture for a more comfortable fit.

Do not accept bargain reconstruction.

You get what you pay for. Cheap dentures rarely fit and can cause damage to the gum and bone tissue. If you are not sure which treatment plan is right for you, get a second opinion from another dentist. It is worth the fee for a consultation and examination to make the right decision.

Implants have been very successful in restoring debilitated mouths.

Ask your dentist if implants are feasible in your particular restoration.

THERE ARE MANY TYPE OF IMPLANTS AND IMPLANT CONSTRUCTION:

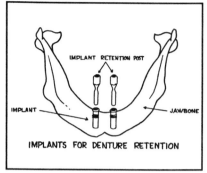

Figure 30A

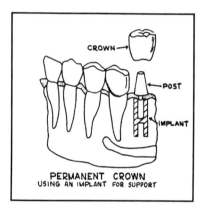

Figure 30B

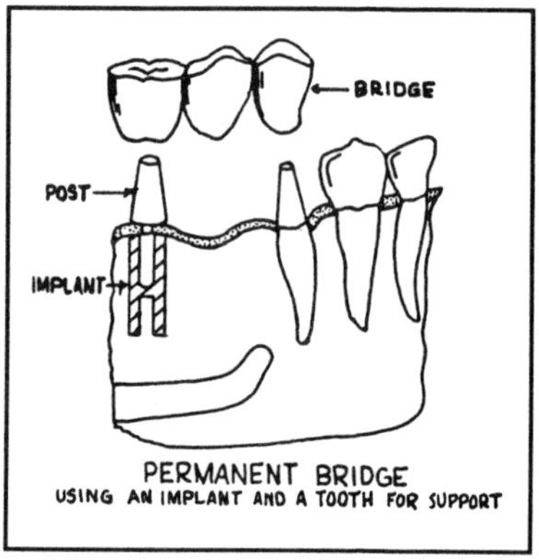

Figure 30C

More about dentures.

Dentures are one way to replace teeth that have been extracted. These can be partial dentures, replacing several teeth, or full dentures, replacing all of the teeth.

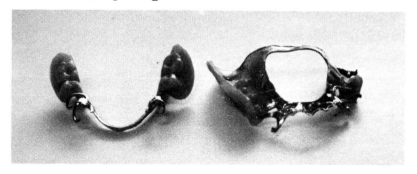

Figure 31 - These are conventional partial dentures with clasps and metal support bars.

Partial Denture Rules

1. Partial dentures should utilize for support, teeth that are, and will remain healthy for many years.
2. Teeth with large fillings, and or gum disease should not be used as major supports for partial dentures.
3. If compromised teeth need to be used for support, be certain they are maximally restored. When necessary, gum therapy and crowns help stabilize the supporting teeth . This should be done before a partial denture is constructed.
4. Partial dentures can be designed for future tooth loss if the patient does not want teeth extracted unless absolutely necessary. These are called transitional partial dentures.

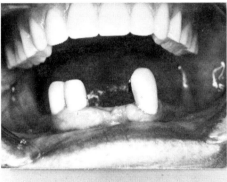

Three precision crowns

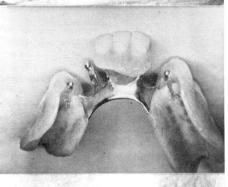

Precision denture

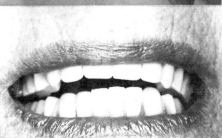

Denture in place

Figure 32 - Three crowns connect to a precision appliance for a comfortable fit.

5. Often, partial dentures can be designed with precision attachments such as magnets, springs, and hinges. These unique attachments will usually enable the partial denture to fit better and last longer.
6. Partial dentures should not have excessive movement during function. Excessive movement will cause the supporting teeth to loosen and hasten their destruction.
7. Partial dentures should not be excessively tight. This strain on the supporting teeth will lead to the failure of this denture.
8. The bite should feel comfortable. All of the teeth should function in unison. No single tooth should be burdened with all of the chewing forces.
9. The gum tissue should not be irritated by the partial denture. Long term gum irritation can be very destructive to the gum and the supporting bone.
10. If you have an ill fitting partial denture, pinpoint the problem to minimize guesswork on the part of the dentist.
11. Partial dentures require extra special maintenance. Frequent rinsing with a pre-rinse and brushing of the supporting teeth is necessary to remove additional plaque buildup, along with frequent cleanings by the dental hygienist. The partial dentures must be removed in order to effectively clean all the areas of these teeth. The partial denture must also be rinsed and brushed in order to insure its longevity.

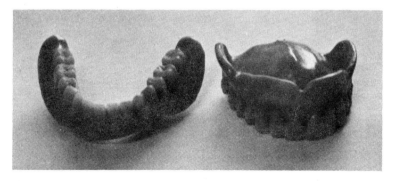

Figure 33 - Full dentures rely on the gum, bone, and muscles for support and retention

Full Denture Rules

1. Full dentures utilize the jaw bone, which is covered by gum tissue, for support. Other oral tissues such as lips, vestibule, and muscles are used to keep the denture from loosening.

2. The patient needs to realize that these are artificial, man made teeth. It is their responsibility to make them work properly.

3. It may be necessary at times to alter ones eating habits when dentures are used. Cutting food into smaller pieces, chewing evenly on both sides, using side teeth for biting into hard foods such as apples, are ways to continue eating foods previously enjoyed. Actively stimulating oral muscles will prevent the dentures from loosening or dislodging. Denture adhesives can be used for additional retention.

4. Sore spots and ill fitting dentures should not be ignored. These problems will cause excessive wear on the supporting bones and gums. This can cause eventual destruction of these tissues and make future dentures more difficult to construct.

5. Ill-fitting dentures can often be repaired by a simple process called relining. This usually requires the patient to be without the denture for twelve to twenty four hours. The newly relined denture should fit comfortably.

6. When dentures are being constructed, a *duplicate* (extra) set can be made at the same time. There is very little extra work involved and they cost considerably less than the original set. This duplicate (transitional) denture can be used as an immediate denture (remove teeth and insert the denture the same day). In three months (after complete healing) the original denture can be relined to fit perfectly. The transitional denture then becomes an extra set There is much security gained from the knowledge that you have an extra set of dentures. You will never be without teeth again. Ask your dentist about this exciting duplicate denture technique.

7. If you have very little bone to support a denture, there are dental procedures that may make denture wearing easier for you.

   A. Vestibuloplasty - Gum tissue can be removed,

replaced, or transposed to enable a denture to seat better in the mouth. This procedure is usually performed by an oral surgeon.

B. Ridge Augmentation - An oral surgeon can replace lost bone tissue by grafting artificial bone into a certain area. For extreme cases of bone loss, a piece of hip bone can be utilized for augmentation.

C. Implants - This is the wave of the future. These may be used for upper and or lower dentures. A periodontist or oral surgeon can often place the implant into the bone that you have left. Your general dentist can then build a new denture utilizing the implant for support retention.

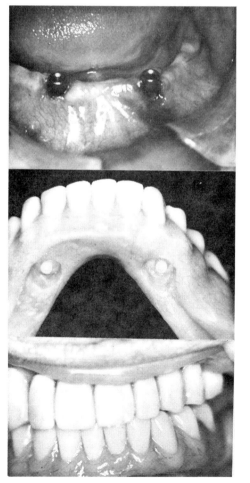

Two implants in the lower jaw.

A denture with implant retention balls inserted.

The denture is in the mouth and stable.

Figure 34.

A word of caution.

I have been to several nursing homes and have seen patients whose dental chewing apparatus has been completely destroyed. These patients could not eat comfortably or adequately, thus depriving their bodies of needed nutrients. I believe this dental destruction hastened the demise of these patients. Please obtain a comfortable chewing apparatus before your body turns the corner down the long road of life.

CHAPTER 17

Questions and Answers

"I keep six honest serving men (they taught me all I knew). Their
names are What and Why and When and How and Where and Who"
Rudyard Kipling 1902

'Why, when and how' are music to my ears. When patients ask questions, they care. If patients care, I can educate them, and it makes my job easier. If I can enlighten them to an understanding of what is happening, and how I intend to treat problems, I may prevent a problem from happening again.

Ask questions. Allow your dentist to educate you as well as treat you. The education is free and may save you from treatment of another problem later on.

The following is a list of the most commonly asked questions and some very short answers:

- *Will this dental treatment hurt*

With modern techniques and gentle care, there is no reason to feel any pain with standard dental treatment.

- *Do you have to drill?*

Usually, in order to remove the decayed portion of an unhealthy tooth and stop further destruction of that tooth, the dental drill must be used. New techniques are being developed which may lessen the amount of drilling necessary for cavity preparation.

- *Do you have to use a needle?*

If the dentist feels as though the procedure might be uncomfortable, the use of local anesthetics will usually be recommended. Local anesthetics will numb the area that is being treated and you should not feel any pain.

- *Why is the needle so long? Does it hurt?*

The length is necessary to reach far back into the mouth. The entire needle does not go into the gum tissue. There is no need to feel the needle with liquid pre-numbing solutions, ultra thin needles, and good techniques. Anesthetic placement can almost always be applied without pain or discomfort.

- Are X-rays necessary?

Yes. In order for a dentist to properly assess, diagnose, and treat your particular dental situation, a full set of X-rays is usually necessary.

- Why?

Very often decay occurs in areas between the teeth where the dentist cannot see. X-rays are necessary for early detection of these lesions. Abscesses, cysts, extra teeth, defects, fractures, and certain cancers can also be detected with dental X-rays.

- Isn't radiation harmful?

With modern machines, fast film, paralleling devices and lead shields, the amount of radiation received is minimal.

- How often should X-rays be taken?

A full series should be taken periodically or as your dentist deems necessary. A panoramic X-ray should also be considered periodically. This type of X-ray will show the entire dental architecture on one X-ray film.

- When is the best age for my child to see the dentist?

As a general rule, by the time the child has reached age 3, he or she should have had at least one dental examination.

- How is the pre–brushing rinse different from mouthwashes?

The pre–brushing rinses use surfactant technology to physically remove some plaque and loosen the remainder to make brushing more effective. Mouthwashes inhibit plaque formation by killing germs that cause plaque, but they aren't designed to *remove* plaque.

- Is fluoride really necessary?

Yes. Consult with your dentist to determine the proper fluoride levels for you and your family.

- What if my child swallows excessive amounts of stannous fluoride rinse?

If the child swallows more than one ounce, have him or her drink several glasses of milk then call your physician for further advice.

- What is the best toothpaste?

You should feel free to choose any toothpaste that is accepted by the American Dental Association (A.D.A.).

- Do you have to use toothpaste?

The physical action of brushing your teeth will remove much

of the plaque that causes decay. Toothpaste aids in the removal of plaque. Toothpaste also freshens your breath and coats the teeth with an additional layer of fluoride.

- What causes cavities?

When food breaks down, residual sugars are left on the teeth. Bacteria which are always present in the mouth, combine with these sugars and form a sticky substance called plaque. This plaque adheres to certain areas of the teeth. The bacteria within the plaque produce an acid waste which demineralizes and can subsequently destroy the tooth. This destruction is known as a cavity.

- How come some people never get cavities?

Some people are just lucky. Their tooth composition and oral bacteria makeup are not conducive to dental breakdown. Other people work hard at good dental care. These people effectively eliminate dental disease by proper diet, proper and regular brushing, flossing, and periodic dental check-ups.

- Are professional dental cleanings necessary?

Yes. Even the best rinsers, brushers and flossers miss cleaning certain areas. Plaque remains in those areas and will harden and form calculus. Only your dentist or hygienist can remove the plaque and calculus with special techniques and instruments.

- What else can happen besides cavities if plaque is not removed from my teeth?

If plaque remains, it will harden into calculus and will promote considerable breakdown of the tooth and supporting structures (gums and bone).

- What is this supporting tissue breakdown?

Periodontal disease (gum disease or pyorrhea).

- What is so bad about periodontal disease?

Periodontal disease is usually not painful or noticeable to the patient until the latter stages of the disease. In short, what happens is this. The plaque slowly erodes the gum and bone which holds the teeth tightly in place. The gums bleed, the teeth become loose and bad breath can result. If the patient does not heed these early warning signals, the destruction continues until the teeth become so loose and uncomfortable that they must be removed.

- If I have periodontal disease, will I lose all of my teeth?

Without early diagnosis and treatment of periodontal disease, you can lose many or all of your teeth. With proper treatment, many or all of your teeth can be saved.

- Can certain drugs cause dental problems?

Yes. Dilantin can cause gingival hypertrophy which is a gum problem. Antidepressants can cause dry mouth, xerostomia, which can lead to a gum problem and tooth decay. Tetracycline, an antibiotic, can cause stained permanent teeth if it is taken early in life between the ages of one and five. Your dentist should be made aware of any drugs that you are taking.

- Can certain diseases cause dental problems?

Yes. Diabetes will often accelerate periodontal distruction. Ask your dentist if your particular disease is associated with possible dental problems.

- If a tooth is lost, is it really necessary to replace it?

Yes. A properly functioning dentition is a necessary ingredient to having a healthy body. Losing an important functional piece of the oral makeup such as a tooth, creates disharmony within the system. The other teeth must work harder, drifting and shifting occur, chewing patterns are altered, and the masticatory system is headed for further breakdown. To prevent further and more complicated problems, certain lost teeth need to be replaced. However, teeth with no functional or aesthetic value such as the wisdom teeth, can be removed without replacement. This will not cause any damage to the system.

- Can an infected tooth be saved?

At times by removing the infected portion of the tooth, the pulp, the tooth can be saved. This is called root canal therapy. You and your dentist should decide if this treatment is right for you.

- Is it painful?

Usually an infected tooth causes pain. The treatment to save the tooth is usually not painful.

- How much would it cost to completely restore a broken down mouth?

The cost will depend upon the amount of dental destruction and the type of reconstruction that is performed.

- How long will good dental care last?

With quality dental treatment, proper maintenance on your part, and routine dental checkups and cleanings, your oral masticatory system can last a lifetime.

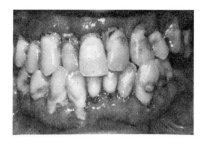 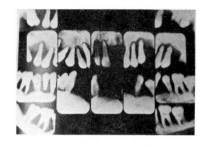

This photograph shows advanced gum disease. Many of these teeth will be lost soon.

This x-ray shows that there is no bone left to support the remaining teeth. All of these teeth must be removed.

Figure 37 - Gum irritation and inflammation can lead to gum, bone, and tooth destruction.

Invest in your health. Maintain and if possible, improve the quality of your teeth and overall oral complex. The benefits you will receive will be well worth the investment.

"Tooth loss is not a normal process of aging. It is caused by neglect." - M. R. 1984

CHAPTER 18

Maximizing Your Dental Dollar

"If you think you can, or can't, you're right.."
A.N. 1985

Quality dental care can be affordable to everyone and should be an integral part of each family's budget. The cost of the treatment may vary. This Chapter explains what you can do to increase the quality and decrease the cost of the dental care you receive.

• Don't wait until you have dental pain to see the dentist. Recognize the early symptoms of dental problems and make your dentist aware of these potential problem areas. Early detection of a problem will enable you to avoid an unpleasant and costly episode in the future.

• Have an overall assessment of your total oral masticatory system, (a thorough examination by the dentist).

• Have a professional dental cleaning at least twice a year. Perform proper brushing and flossing routinely.

• Inform your dentist of any of the following problems: Food catches, rough edges of teeth or fillings, hot, cold, or sweet sensitive areas, pressure sensitive teeth, bleeding gums, foul odor or taste coming from a tooth, loose fillings, loose teeth, persistent sores or lesions, headaches and neckaches, tooth grinding problems etc. Inform the dentist of areas that you wish him or her to examine more closely. This will usually lead to early diagnosis and treatment of a problem.

• Ask to see the X-ray and the teeth with a mirror, that the dentist will be working on. Your interest and concern can be an inspiration which will increase the dentist's quest for excellence when he or she works on your teeth.

• Ask to see the restored teeth when the dentist has completed his/her work. Compliment him or her if you are satisfied. When a patient appreciates what is done for him or her, future work is usually performed with an extra touch of quality.

• If the filling feels high, rough or out of place, tell the dentist. Let him or her adjust it for you before you leave the office. You will save yourself a return trip and avoid the temporary discomfort of an unfinished filling.

- If possible, schedule your appointments for the morning. This time of day is usually less busy in the dental office.

- If you can handle it mentally and physically, ask your dentist to schedule one long appointment rather than several short appointments for fillings. His/her time with you will be more productive.

- If you must change your appointment time, call the office at least 48 hours in advance. If you do not intend to keep your appointment, that time spot can be used for another patient.

- Do not avoid necessary dental treatment simply because it is not covered by your dental insurance policy. If your car needed brakes, you would spend the money for new brakes. If your tooth needs a cap, get a cap. Do not let an insurance policy dictate the quality of care that you receive.

- Have a general idea what your dental insurance covers. Do not assume that because you have insurance you will no longer have any dental bills.

- After your dental cleaning, schedule your next cleaning in advance. This will force you to seek regular dental care. Remember, proper maintenance is the key to saving money in the future. You will also be able to reserve the time of your choice.

- Establish a good rapport with the receptionist. She is a powerful friend to have on your side in the event of an emergency, billing error, scheduling or insurance problems.

- Send a holiday card to your dentist and staff. You can even bring in some homemade cookies or jam for them. Try to be 'that nice patient'. If you are nice to others, they will be nice to you.

- Refer new patients to your dentist if you are happy with his/her work. A referring patient is a special patient in the eyes of the dentist (thanks Sue Locasto, Terry Kovlak and many more).

- Make the work easier on yourself and your dentist:
  1. Sit still, open wide, adjust your head and body so that it is comfortable for him or her to work.
  2. Sit up and rinse as little as possible. Each time you move, it breaks the flow of treatment and the dentist's concentration.
  3. Try to relax and let him or her perform the dental work that is necessary. By reducing your anxiety, the dentist will be able to treat your problem quickly and easily.
  4. The easier it is for the dentist to work, the better the treatment will be.

• Proper maintenance of your teeth is the real key to saving money on dental care. If the treatment is done properly the first time, and you take care of what has been done, you will increase the longevity of your oral health.

The Cost of Dental Care

• Since each tooth has five sides to it, the more sides of a tooth that need restoration, the more the filling for that tooth will cost.

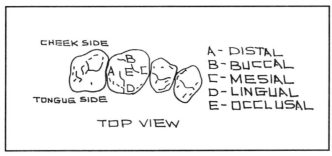

Figure 39A - Each side of a tooth has a name.

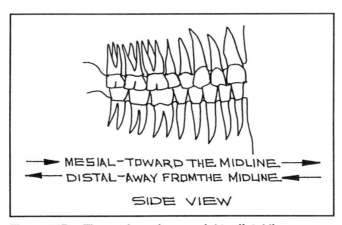

Figure 39B - The teeth are in a mesial to distal line.

• The cost of crowns may vary depending upon the type of material used. The least expensive are stainless steel and plastic, while the more expensive are porcelain, gold, and the new synthetics.

• The longevity of a crown's existence depends upon:
1. The health of the tooth and the supporting tissue upon which the crown is placed.
2. The fit between the crown and the tooth.
3. The home care habits of the patient.

4. The cement which is used.

5. The material of the crown.

• The cost of a root canal may vary depending upon the number of canals within the tooth. The central incisor has one canal, the first bicuspid has two canals, molars have three or more.

• The cost for an extraction may vary depending on the difficulty of the extraction. Simple extractions are less expensive.

• The cost for partial and complete dentures may vary depending on the foundation of the remaining teeth and bone support.

• Whatever the cost for reconstruction, the basic rule is: **Do it once, do it right.** Early detection and treatment of dental problems can save you money. It will also enable you to avoid painful experiences in the future. Do not put off until tomorrow what you can do today.

QUICK REFERENCE FOR PAIN DIAGNOSIS

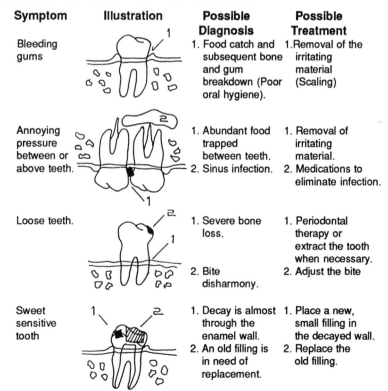

Symptom	Illustration	Possible Diagnosis	Possible Treatment
Bleeding gums		1. Food catch and subsequent bone and gum breakdown (Poor oral hygiene).	1. Removal of the irritating material (Scaling)
Annoying pressure between or above teeth.		1. Abundant food trapped between teeth. 2. Sinus infection.	1. Removal of irritating material. 2. Medications to eliminate infection.
Loose teeth.		1. Severe bone loss. 2. Bite disharmony.	1. Periodontal therapy or extract the tooth when necessary. 2. Adjust the bite
Sweet sensitive tooth		1. Decay is almost through the enamel wall. 2. An old filling is in need of replacement.	1. Place a new, small filling in the decayed wall. 2. Replace the old filling.

(Continued)

QUICK REFERENCE FOR PAIN DIAGNOSIS (Continued)

Symptom	Illustration	Possible Diagnosis	Possible Treatment
Cold sensitive tooth.	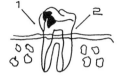	1. Decay is thru the outer tooth wall. 2. Gum recession has caused gum-line sensitivity.	1. Place a new filling in the tooth 2. Place a liner or plastic layer over the sensitive area
Hot sensitive tooth	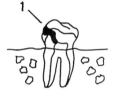	1. Decay is near the pulp tissue.	1. Place a filling with a medicated liner or place a temporary filling or perform root canal therapy.
Pain on pressure	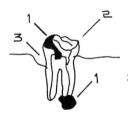	1. Decay is in the pulp chamber and an abscess is forming. 2. There is a fracture line within the tooth. 3. The tooth is periodontally compromised.	1. Root canal therapy or extract the tooth. 2. Crown the tooth for for support, root canal therapy, or extraction. 3. Periodontal therapy.

CHAPTER 19

X-rays—
Dental Radiographs—
A Pictorial Analysis

A picture is worth a thousand words

X-rays (Radiographs) are an integral part of the dental diagnostic procedure. If it were not for the aid of the dental radiograph, dental problems would often remain undetected. Undetected problems grow and become large problems later on. Even though x-rays do not present every aspect of the potential problem, they should be taken and observed prior to most dental treatments. Unfortunately the dental radiograph is a two dimensional picture of a three dimensional object. It may often be necessary to take several radiographs of the same problem area from different angles. This comparative x-ray technique will more closely represent a three dimensional tooth. This will aid in the diagnosis and treatment of the problem.

The following is a brief overview of reading dental radiographs. This should help you to understand your particular dental situation when your dentist shows you x-rays:

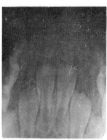

The baby teeth are visible inside the mouth as the permanent teeth develop under the bone.

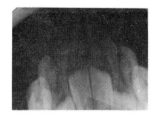

The baby teeth resorb as the permanent teeth continue to develop.

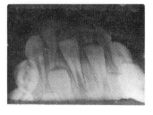

One baby tooth is lost as one permanent tooth becomes visible inside the mouth.

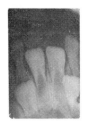

The permanent teeth develop as some baby teeth have already been lost.

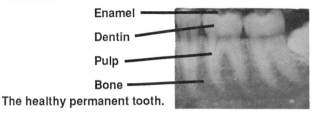

Enamel

Dentin

Pulp

Bone

The healthy permanent tooth.

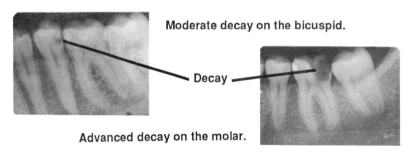

Moderate decay on the bicuspid.

Decay

Advanced decay on the molar.

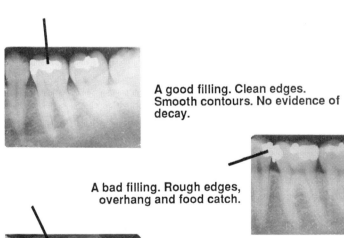

A good filling. Clean edges. Smooth contours. No evidence of decay.

A bad filling. Rough edges, overhang and food catch.

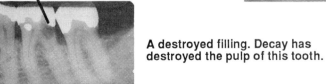

A destroyed filling. Decay has destroyed the pulp of this tooth.

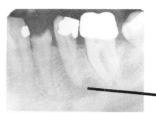

The pulp tissue in this tooth has died and has caused an abscess to form. Pain, swelling and mobility are some possible symptoms of this problem.

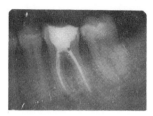

This tooth has been saved by root canal therapy. The infected nerve tissue has been removed and a filler material has been placed into the pulp chamber (root canal).

A permanent bridge.

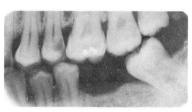

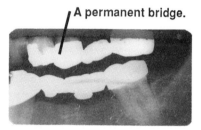

If a tooth is lost, several problems can follow: Decay of the bicuspid is probably due to the drifting of the teeth as caused by the loss of the lower molars.

If lost teeth are replaced early, future destruction can be avoided.

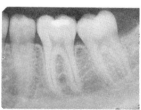

Healthy gum tissue is supported by healthy bone.

Bone contour is flat and level.

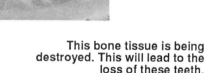

This bone tissue is being destroyed. This will lead to the loss of these teeth.

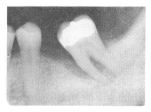

This bone is in terrible shape. The tooth is probably not salvageable and will have to be removed.

CHAPTER 20

The Psychodental Transformation (Cosmetic Dentistry)

Let a smile be your umbrella.

Every person has a perception of self that greatly affects the way that they interact with the rest of the world. This perception is known as one's self-image. If you look marvelous, your chances of feeling marvelous are greatly improved.

Through the art of cosmetic dental reconstruction we are able to alter your dental appearance (your smile). Most often a persons self-image is positively transformed with their improved esthetics. They will look better, and subsequently feel better about themselves. I have labeled this occurrence The Psychodental Transformation.

The following pictorial review should give you a general idea of the potential transformations that can occur with improved dental esthetics.

Children

The child's developing speech patterns, smile habits, and self-image are often affected by his or her dental appearance. A psychodental transformation at this early stage in life may greatly enhance the child's developing psychological makeup.

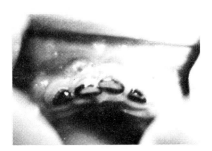

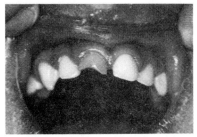

Figure 40 A - *Baby bottle syndrome.* **This child is three years old. These teeth must be removed and the child may never smile.**

Figure 40 B - **There are potential physical and psychological hazards to leaving this situation untreated. The dark, traumatized tooth needs dental care.**

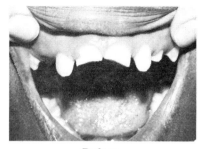 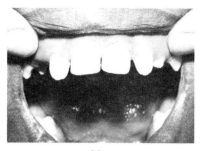

| Before | After |

Figure 40C - This traumatic injury can be easily treated through the art of cosmetic bonding

Adolescents

The dental adolescent (age 7-16), is undergoing a natural dental transformation. They begin to lose their baby teeth, show their permanent teeth, and alter their facial jaw structure. In conjunction with these alterations, their self-image evolves from a child to that of a young adult. With the aid of certain creative dental techniques, their dental esthetics can be improved. This improved smile will certainly enhance the adolescent's self-image.

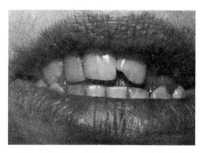 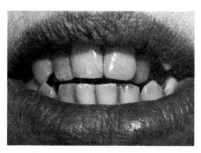

| Before | After |

Figure 41A - A pin build-up and bonding technique was necessary to restore this child's smile.

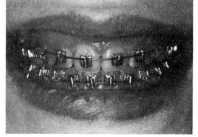

Figure 41B - Orthodontic therapy is a true creative art form. The psychodental transformations obtained from the procedure are remarkable.

Adults

The psychodental transformation of the adult is usually a dramatic and exciting occurrence for both the dentist and the patient. With the use of modern creative dental techniques and materials, we can transform the dental appearance (the smile) from dull to dazzling. Let the imagination of both you and your dentist transform your smile into one that you will be proud of.

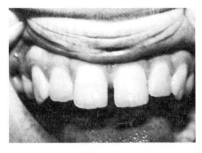 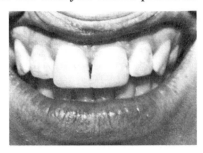

Before   *After*

Figure 42A - Office veneer bonding techniques can solve stain and contour problems.

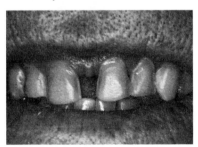 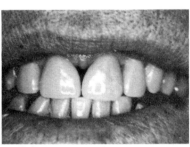

Before   *After*

Figure 42B - More advanced (lab) bonding techniques are necessary for larger alterations.

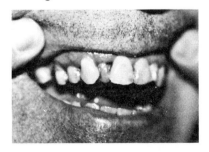 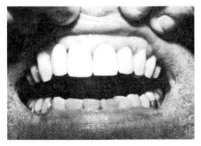

Before   *After*

Figure 42C - Instant orthodontics. Esthetic, health, and functional improvement can be achieved through modern dental techniques. (One tooth has been removed and a permanent bridge has been inserted.)

Note: Bleaching (whitening), a new and exciting cosmetic technique, is now available for the general public.

Seniors

Seniors look around you. Do some of your friends appear older or younger than their chronological age? Take a second look at these individuals. Evaluate their dental health and how often they smile. I believe that you will see a definite correlation between individuals with a healthy, pleasing smile and their youthful attitudes towards life.

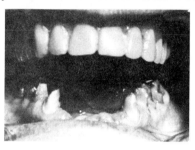
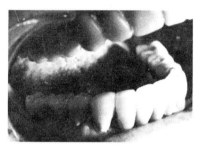

Before *After*

Figure 43A - Implants have been utilized on the lower right to facilitate a permanently cemented bridge for this patient.

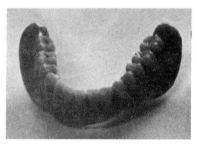
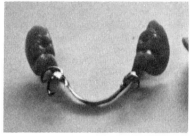

Figure 43B - A regular denture replaces all of the missing teeth.

Figure 43C - A partial denture replaces several or many missing teeth.

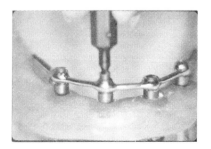
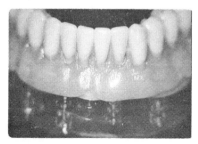

Figure 43D - An implant retained denture can permanently replace many or all missing teeth. The implants seen here can be constructed upon for permanent tooth replacement.

CHAPTER 21

Nutrition

"Eat to live, and not live to eat"
Benjamin Franklin 1733

What good is a great set of teeth if the rest of the body is falling to pieces? Dentists are becoming more aware of the need to treat the entire person rather than an isolated pearly white in the corner of the mouth.

There are many excellent books on nutrition. Check with your physician or dentist to see which one he or she recommends. The nutrition chart on the following pages briefly outlines the need for vitamins and minerals.

There are four basic food groups.

They are dairy, meat, vegetable/fruit and bread/cereal. A well–balanced meal should contain a reasonable blend from the basic food groups. When a meal contains a proper mix of these foods, the nutritional needs of the individual are usually satisfied.

The preparation of certain foods will often reduce or even eliminate the vitamins and minerals that may have been provided by that food. If the juices of the food are lost while cooking (boiled and drained), it is likely that the vitamins and minerals have been lost also.

Vitamin supplements

Vitamin supplements (vitamin pills) are recommended if you believe that your daily eating habits do not furnish you with enough vitamins and minerals. Consult your physician, dentist, nutritionist, or chiropractor. They will recommend a high quality vitamin/mineral supplement for you.

Nutrition Chart

Vitamin or Mineral	Food Source
A	Vegetables, fruits, dairy products, beef
B 1 Thyamine	Fish, meat, wheat germ
B 2 Riboflavin	Dairy, eggs, brewers yeast
B 3	Vegetables, meat, dairy, poultry
B 5	Eggs, vegetables, fish
B 6 Pyridoxine	Dairy, vegetables, liver
B 12 Cobolamin	Beef, dairy, eggs, fish
C	Fruits, some vegetables
D	Eggs, fish, dairy, sunshine
K	Vegetables

Function	Deficiency Symptoms
Helps to form bones, teeth, hair and skin. Used for night vision, tissue growth and repair	Allergies, night blindness, fatigue, itching, burnining eyes and dry skin
Helps with digestion, nervous system functions and cardiac functions	Constipation, depression, nervousness, loss of appetite
Used for antibody and red blood cell formation	Cataracts; itchy, burning eyes; cracks in the corner of the mouth; red, sore tongue
Used for nervous system growth; needed for maintenance of healthy skin, tongue and hair	Mouth sores; bad mouth odor; muscle aches
Needed for antibody formation and stress resistance	Hair loss, early aging, respiratory infections, diarrhea
Used for food metabolism, ion balance for the nervous system, and antibody formation	Loss of muscle control, nervousness, depression, anemia and arthritis
Necessary for red blood cell formation, metabolism, and a healthy nervous system	Anemia, weakness, nervousness, poor appetite
Needed for infection resistance, formation of bones, teeth, and red blood cells	Anemia, bleeding gums, slow wound healing, frequent colds and infections
Needed for heralthy bone, nervous system and tooth formation	Burning sensation of the mouth, nervousness, soft teeth and bones, weakness and insomnia
Needed for proper blood clotting	Nosebleeds, diarrhea, bleeding problems

Nutrition Chart

Vitamin or Mineral	Food Source
E	Vegetables, eggs and meats
Calcium	Dairy, some fish and meats
Copper	Vegetables and some meats and fish
Iron	Liver, fish, eggs and meat
Potassium	Fruits and vegetables
Sodium	Dairy and some fish
Iodine	Iodized salt, fish
Zinc	Meats, vegetables, fish

Function	*Deficiency Symptoms*
Needed for blood cholesterol reduction and enhancement of other vitamins' functions	Dry hair, heart disease, elevated cholesterol levels
Needed for bone and tooth formation, muscle reactions, and blood clotting	Muscle cramps, tooth decay, nervousness
Needed for red blood cell formation, bone formation, and healing processes	Anemia, weakness, and a tendancy to have skin irritations
It is a main component of the red blood cells	Weakness, fatigue, shortness of breath
Needed for proper nervous system functioning	Poor reflexes, constipation, heart problems
Needed for proper muscle contractions and nervous system reactions	Poor muscle tone, poor muscle control and nervous system response
Needed for metabolism regulation	Dry hair, nervousness, obesity
Needed for proper wound healing	Loss of taste, fatigue, slow wound healing

Dieting to lose weight is overrated.

If you believe that you need to lose weight to improve your health (physical and emotional), be sure to consult your physician first. Do not rush into the latest fad diet, diet group, or pills. The secret to looking and feeling trim (healthy) is centered within an individual's mind. One must first *clarify* the reason for losing weight before any true long term weight loss can be achieved. Support groups are highly recommended once you have decided the need and true inner reason for losing excess weight.

Daily exercise

Daily exercise is also necessary for the body to maintain a high level of efficiency. Even a short 1/2 hour daily warm-up exercise will add years and energy to your life. Exercise can be as little as stretching and light aerobics or as complex as Tae Quan Do.

The time you dedicate to your body can also be dedicated to your mind

During your daily routine, do not allow worldly problems to enter your thought patterns. You deserve this time to free your mind of the problems of day to day life. They will still be there after your exercise, so do not let them ruin that special time that you have graciously granted yourself.

Your body is the only one you have. You are responsible for the care and maintenance of it. Be good to it, and it will be good to you.

CHAPTER 22

The Reference Chapter:

What Is It?

"Every man is fully satisfied that there is such a thing as truth, or he would not ask questions".
C.S. Pierce 1958

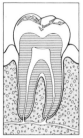

- **Tooth** - a vital part of your body which decreases food particle size while chewing.
- **Gums** - a layer of tissue which covers the jawbone.
- **Bone** - that which supports the teeth.

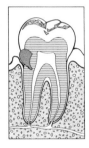

- **Plaque** - a sticky substance containing food and bacteria. (Plaque causes tooth decay and periodontal disease.)

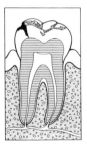

- **Caries (cavity)** - a dental disease characterized by a progressive destruction of the tooth surface and core.

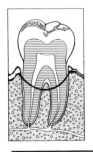

- **Periodontal disease (pyorrhea)** - destruction of the gum and bone tissue which will lead to tooth loss.

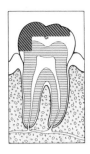

- **Filling** - a plastic, porcelain, or metal restoration placed in a tooth after decay has been removed.

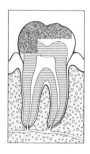

- **Temporary medicated filling** - a medication placed in the tooth to calm an irritated pulp (nerve). This is done if the cavity is deep in an attempt to avoid root canal treatment.

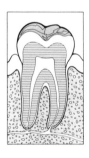

- **Laminates** - porcelain or resin like coating which is bonded to the tooth. This can alter the color and shape of the tooth.
- **Sealant** - a plastic like coating which is bonded to teeth to prevent decay.

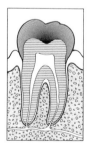

- **Cap (crown)** - a protective restoration which covers a tooth.

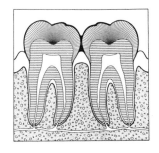

- **Splint** - a way of connecting periodontally loose teeth.

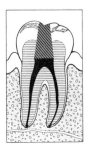

- **Equilibration** - the adjustment of teeth to properly align the bite which may help to eliminate a T. M. J. problem.
- **Nightguard** - a plastic or rubber like appliance which can lessen the destructive effects caused by clenching and grinding.

- **Root canal treatment** - the removal of the dead or dying pulpal tissue.

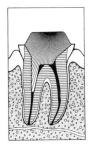

- **Post** - a way to rebuild the base of a tooth after a root canal has been completed. A crown should be placed over the post.

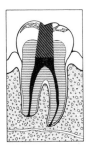

- **Apicoectomy** - the removal of the tip of the root and the remaining residual infection. This may be necessary if the root canal therapy has been unsuccessful.

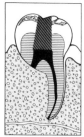

• **Hemisection** - the removal of one of the roots of a multi- rooted tooth.

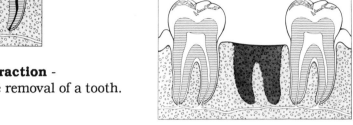

• **Extraction** -
the removal of a tooth.

• **Bridge** - a way of permanently replacing a lost tooth before further destruction occurs. The neighboring teeth are utilized for support.

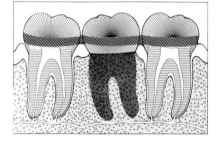

• **Bonded Maryland bridge** - a bridge which is bonded to neighboring teeth. This is not possible in some cases.
• **Partial removable denture** - a way to replace several or many missing teeth.
• **Precision Attachment (retained partial denture)** - An esthetic partial denture retained by hidden connectors instead of visible clasps (hooks).
• **Complete denture** - a way to replace all of the missing teeth. Dentures are held in place by suction, a tight fit, muscle tone, and/or adhesives.
• **Implant** - a metal insert placed into the bone of a toothless area. This can be used to rebuild the masticatory system. A bridge, partial denture, or even a full denture can be constructed over an implant. This will improve function, aesthetics and comfort in most cases. This is the wave of the future for dental reconstruction.
• **Tissue graft** - replacement of bone or gum tissue where necessary.

CHAPTER 23

The T.M.J.
(Temporomandibular Joint)

*The hinge joint that connects the
upper and lower jaws*

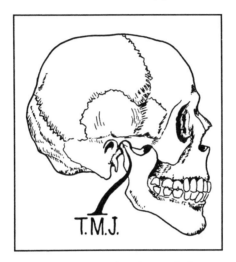

**The T.M.J. is the most complex bone joint connection in
the body. It consists of:**

- Two sets of bones, the mandible and the temporal
  bones.
- One set of articulating discs.
- Seven sets of muscles for each joint, which must
  function harmoniously.
- Two joints on opposite sides of the mandible which
  must function harmoniously.
- As many as 32 teeth which determine the T.M.J.'s
  position while chewing.
- A unique blood supply system which allows for a
  wide range of motion within the T.M.J.
- A nerve relay system that coordinates the entire oral
  complex.

The joint is designed to move in almost any possible direction. Excessive deviant motions of the mandible can cause a
T.M.J. problem.

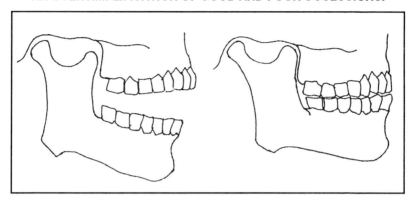

Open   Closed

With a *good* occlusion (bite), the condylar head (the movable portion of the jaw apparatus) is within the socket and is unstressed in both the open and closed positions.

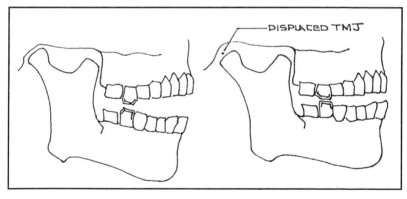

Open   Closed

With a malocclusion, when closed, the teeth are hitting in an uneven fashion. This forces the mandible to move to a position which creates excessive stress upon the T.M.J. complex.

Constant unnecessary pressure in the joint area can lead to:

• Muscle spasms of the joint area.
   • Pain and limited jaw opening.
   • Headaches in the temple and back of neck areas.
   • Arthritis of the joint.
   • Excessive wear and eventual destruction of the T. M. J.
   • Sensitive teeth.
   • Fractures of teeth that are causing the disharmony.
   • Loosening of teeth and destruction of bone that supports the malpositioned tooth.

Possible solutions to a T.M.J. problem may include:

- Eliminate the habit which activates the occlusal dishar-mony. This may eliminate the problem. Habits may include clenching, grinding, nail biting,unbalanced chewing, night grinding, lip biting, and nervous twitches. If a person is confronted with the fact that he or she has a destructive habit, he or she may be able to stop the habit.
- A bite guard can be constructed to help stop the de-structive habit of grinding and clenching.
- Muscle relaxants may be necessary to relieve the muscle spasm.
- If necessary, equilibration of the dental arch may create occlusal harmony. This involves selective grinding of the offending teeth (the ones that are hitting out of unison with the others). Several visits may be necessary to fully adjust the bite.
- The occlusion (bite) can be rebuilt to create a harmoni-ous biting surface that coincides with the movements of the T.M.J. This internal reconstruction may include caps, bridges, or partial dentures.
- New, properly aligned dentures may be necessary for denture patients with T.M.J. pain.
- Surgery of the joint area may be necessary in extreme cases of T.M.J. disorders.
- Chiropractic, orthopedic and podiatric physicians may need to be included in a multi–disciplined approach to cure a T.M.J. problem.

The T.M.J. is instrumental for the proper functioning of the chewing system.

For a lifetime of healthy eating, it is necessary to maintain this joint in perfect working order. Make sure that your dentist examines this joint area at least once a year.

Find the cause and you will find the cure.

The cause of a TMJ problem is usually related to stress and anxiety. Relax and stop destroying your TMJ. Although the assistance of a dentist may be necessary, the balance of TMJ cure rests within the patient's ability to "mellow out."

"Be patient today so you won't be a patient in the hospital tomorrow."
Mr. Woods 1989

CHAPTER 24

Choosing the Right Dentist For You

A man's a man who looks a man
right between the eyes.

Most people already have a dentist. Whether they go to him or her often enough is another story. Before deciding what qualities to look for in a new dentist, let's assess your present oral caretaker...

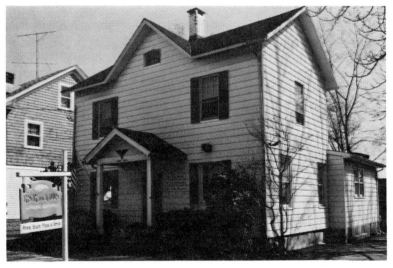

Figure 44 -
YES/NO

     _ _ Do you like your dentist?
     _ _ Do you trust your dentist?
     _ _ Do you think that the dental work (fillings etc.) is of high quality?
     _ _ Does your dentist take continuing education courses?
     _ _ Is the dental office neat and clean?
     _ _ Is your dentist neatly and cleanly dressed?
     _ _ Is your dentist caring and personable?
     _ _ Is the dental staff caring and personable?
     _ _ Does your dentist listen to what you have to say?

___ Does your dentist answer your questions to your satisfaction?

___ Are most of your dental visits painless?

___ Does your dentist and hygienist stress good dental home care?

___ Does your dentist try to insist on proper dental maintenance (cleanings)?

___ Do your dentist's hands feel sturdy and well-positioned when he or she works on your mouth?

___ Are the dental instruments sterilized?

___ Does your dentist feel proud of his/her or her work?

___ Do the fillings your dentist places in your mouth feel smooth and comfortable to bite on?

___ Does your dentist wear gloves?

___ Does your dentist appear 100% alert?

___ Does your dentist treat you as a person and not just another mouth?

___ Is the dental office in a convenient location?

___ Do your dentist's teeth look good?

___ Has your dentist suggested possible reconstruction that you might need?

___ Did your dentist present a total picture of your oral health needs and provide you with alternatives for treatment?
Example: white fillings or silver fillings; fixed or removable bridgework; orthodontics, implants, etc.

___ Do your teeth feel good?

Count up the number of YES answers, and multiply that number by 4. Out of a possible 100 test score, the number you end up with is the grade that your dentist receives on this short assessment exam.

Assuming that most dentists charge about the same, why would anyone go to a dentist who is not at least an 85% quality dentist? I'll tell you why: guilt, fear, and location.

People feel guilty if they go to any dentist other than the one they have already seen, even if they are dissatisfied with him or her. Patients feel a moral obligation to return to the dentist who already has their records and x-rays. They might not return to the dentist until pain occurs rather than switch to a new dentist.

Fear is another reason for sticking with the mediocre dentist. A patient may leave his/her office and not have been hurt too badly. He or she may have felt fairly comfortable, and the filling may only feel sharp on one corner. Had he or she gone to another dentist, things might have been worse.

The convenience of the dentist's location and scheduling hours are very important to most individuals. I realize the importance of this particular reason. However, the easy way is not always the best way.

It is your mouth, and it is up to you to determine the quality of dental treatment that is placed within it. If your dentist got a bad grade, consider visiting another dentist and then revaluate the dental care that you have received. If need be, try a third dentist. If your dentist got a good grade, smile proudly with confidence and stick with him or her.

How to Seek Out The A+ Dentist

1. Ask friends and neighbors who their dentist is. Ask several friends from different areas of the community.
   a. Ask them if they like their dentist and the work he or she does.
   b. Casually look at their teeth and assess the work that has been done.
   c. Ride by the offices of the dentists that have been recommended. Assess the buildings and grounds of their dental homes. A dentist's office is often a reflection of his/her inner self.
   d. Enter into the waiting rooms and talk to the receptionists. Get a feel for the personality of the offices.
2. Ask your doctor or pediatrician whom he or she recommends, then follow steps c and d.
3. Look in the yellow pages. Find several convenient dental locations and then follow steps 1 and 2. Do not believe all of the advertising that you read.
4. Call a specialist such as an oral surgeon, periodontist, or an orthodontist. Tell him or her you are new in town and request the name of a high quality general dentist. Then follow steps c and d.

When changing dentists, follow these guidelines:

If you are new to a community or if you have decided that you must switch dentists, you should follow an organized approach for the continuation of your dental treatment and the transfer of your records.

1. If you want to change dentists, *first* be certain that you are not making a rash decision. Ask yourself to

clarify the reasons for switching. These might include a problem with location (you have moved to another area), the billing system, the office staff, the quality of the dental care, the attitude of the dentist, etc. Once you have focused on the problem, make a sincere effort to resolve it with your present dentist. Many problems can be resolved easily once both parties understand the specifics.

2. Find your new dentist by the techniques stated earlier in this Chapter. Once you have selected a new dentist, call his/her office and make an appointment for consultation or a cleaning and examination. In the case of an emergency (pain), most dentists will be able to see you the day you call.

3. Once you have established an appointment time you can inform the receptionist of the name, address and telephone number of your previous dentist. Ask the receptionist to call and have your x–rays and records sent to the new dentist.

4. You can call your previous dentist and request that the x-rays and a copy of your records be sent to your new dentist: be prepared to provide the receptionist with the name, address and telephone number. This coordinated effort in the transfer of your dental records will improve the chances that they will be present when you go to your first dental visit at the new office.

5. If you have and unpaid bill at your previous dentist, be sure to make arrangements to settle your account before you move or have your records transferred. A relationship with your new dentist should begin with fairness, honesty, respect and an appreciation of the quality health care you will receive.

Do not shop for a dentist solely by comparing fees. Bargain hunting while purchasing parachutes, fire extinguishers, and dental care is foolish.

CHAPTER 25

The Dental Team

"A long pull and a strong pull, and a pull together."
Charles Dickens 1850

The oral complex is probably the most intricate system in the human body. Seven sub-specialty classifications are required within the dental profession. For each sub-specialty classification, an additional two to three years of dental training is necessary after completion of four years of dental school. These sub-specialists in the field of dentistry are instrumental in creating a total dental team. Under the careful management and direction of a general dentist, the necessary specialists can be utilized for your particular dental situation.

The following will briefly outline the complete oral care team.

THE GENERAL DENTIST
- They are trained in all phases of dental care.
- They are licensed to perform all phases of dental care.
- Their specialty is usually diagnosis and treatment planning.
- They know their limitations and will use a specialist when necessary to perform certain procedures.
- They will be the coordinator for dental care if specialists are to be involved.

Their team of specialists consists of:

The Pedodontist-
- Specializes in dental care for children.
- Treats extremely young children (under two).
- Treats problem (extremely fearful) children.
- Treats advanced dental problems (abundant decay).

The Orthodontist-
- Specializes in realigning the teeth with braces.
- They aid in the proper development of jaw relationships and facial contours.

The Oral (Maxilofacial) Surgeon-
- Specializes in major jawbone reconstruction and repair.
- They remove teeth such as wisdom teeth etc.
- They perform implants.

The Endodontist-
- Specializes in performing root canal therapies [the removal of infected tooth tissue (pulp) in order to save the tooth].

The Periodontist-
- Specializes in the treatment of gum disease.
- They reshape the bone which supports the teeth.
- They perform implants

The Prosthodontist-
- Specializes in full mouth reconstruction.

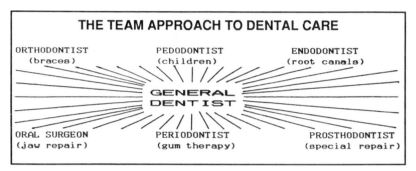

THE TEAM APPROACH TO DENTAL CARE

ORTHODONTIST (braces) — PEDODONTIST (children) — ENDODONTIST (root canals) — GENERAL DENTIST — ORAL SURGEON (jaw repair) — PERIODONTIST (gum therapy) — PROSTHODONTIST (special repair)

Within the dental office is another team of professionals:

The Dental Hygienist
- They work in the General Dentist's office.
- They will question your medical health, and possibly check your blood pressure.
- They are responsible for cleaning plaque and calculus from your teeth.
- They educate patients about teeth and proper brushing and flossing techniques.
- They inform the dentist of possible oral health problems while doing routine cleanings.
- They will take necessary X-rays.

The Dental Receptionist-
- They oversee phone control, appointment setting, billing, insurance, filing, and supply purchasing. They are also responsible for many other tasks.

The Dental Assistant-
- They assist the dentist while working on the patient (four hands are better than two).
- They are responsible for keeping a smooth patient flow, ordering dental supplies, confirming the schedule and innumerable other duties.

The Office Manager-
- They are responsible for running a smooth office .
- They are the coordinator, problem solver and in charge of implementing office policy.

The Dental Laboratory Technician-
- They are responsible for the natural appearance of dental prosthetics taken from impressions made by the dentist.
- They create custom made dental devices such as bridges, dentures, or crowns.

CHAPTER 26

The Dental Insurance Story

"You get what you pay for."
Gabriel Biel 1425–1495

All dental insurance policies are not created equal. There are often misconceptions about what a particular dental insurance plan will pay for. The best way to completely understand your dental insurance coverage is to read the brochure provided by your company. This can be easily obtained from the personnel department. If after scanning the policy, you do not fully understand your coverage, bring the policy to your dentist. His or her office manager or receptionist will be glad to interpret the policy for you.

The information in this chapter will be helpful to you in understanding your dental insurance policy coverage.

Definitions

- *Deductible-* the amount you pay yearly to the dentist before any insurance coverage begins.
- *% Coverage-* this is the percentage of the bill (after the deductible is met) that the insurance company will pay.
- *Yearly maximum-* the total amount of money that your insurance company will pay for dental care each year.
- *Usual and customary-* this is an arbitrary amount for a particular dental service. This dollar amount is established by the insurance company. This amount may not be the actual usual and customary fee charged by dentists in a certain area. This terminology (usual and customary) is an insurance company term which attempts to justify why they did not pay for all of your dental treatment.
- *Not covered-* certain insurance policies do not cover certain dental procedures. This does not mean that these procedures are not necessary. It means that your insurance company has set a limit on the benefits you are able to receive.
- *Riders-* certain policies will cover certain procedures only if you have riders. These are extra insurance bonuses which will usually cover some of the more

involved dental techniques (orthodontics, caps, dentures, gum therapy).

•*Pre–treatment estimate*- assume that the dentist has devised a comprehensive treatment plan for your particular dental situation. To be aware of exactly how much money your insurance company will pay towards this work, a pre-treatment estimate should be sent to the insurance company. This allows all the parties involved to be aware of all of the financial responsibilities before treatment is started.

•*Scheduled benefit amount*- this is a dollar amount that your insurance company will pay for a certain dental procedure. This amount is established by the insurance company. It is often considerably less than what the dentist's fees actually are.

EXAMPLE #1*

Dental Policy: $25 deductible, 100% routine coverage
Rider A: Crowns and dentures 80%

Treatment Plan		Insurance Coverage		Patient Balance
Cleaning &				
X-rays	$ 70	$25 deductible +		
		$45 @ 100% cov.	$ 45	$ 25
2 fillings	100	100% coverage	100	——
1 crown	500	80% coverage	400	100
1 denture	600	80% coverage	480	120
Bill:	$1270	Insurance:	$1025	Patient: $245

EXAMPLE #2*

Dental Policy: $50 deductible, 80% coverage
Rider B: Crowns at 50%, dentures not covered

Treatment Plan		Insurance Coverage		Patient Balance
Cleaning &				
X-rays		$50 deductible +		
		$20 @ 80% cov.	$ 16	$ 54
2 fillings	100	80% coverage	80	20
1 crown	500	50% coverage	250	250
1 denture	600	Not covered	——	600
Bill:	$1270	Insurance:	$346	Patient $924

*These are only examples: The fees and policy descriptions will vary. (1984 fee and insurance company estimate.)

Dental insurance is an insurance agreement between the insurance company and you. You are financially responsible to pay the dentist. Your insurance company is financially responsible to reimburse you for dental expenses you have incurred.

Your dentist may be willing to deal directly with the insurance company. This will relieve you of burdensome paperwork.

You are responsible for whatever the insurance company does not pay towards your dental balance.

You can maximize the amount of money that your insurance pays towards your dental work in the following ways:

• Utilize the dental coverage that is available. If cleanings are covered, make sure that you receive routine cleanings.

• Once the deductible is met, complete all of the necessary dental work (fillings) that the dentist recommends. Try to do that within the dental calendar year. Try not to exceed your yearly maximum.

• If the insurance company is willing to pay $300 towards a $500 crown, get it done. They are giving you money to improve your oral health. Don't pass up a considerable savings on necessary dental work.

• Sometimes (because of the maximum yearly coverage) the insurance company will not cover the cost for the total treatment plan. It is often possible to break the treatment plan into stages. Have some of the dental work done this year and some next year.

If it is necessary to do all the work at once, start in November and complete the project in January. Inquire as to which month your dental benefits begin. It is possible to receive maximum insurance coverage this way.

If your spouse has dental insurance also, both insurances can be utilized (co–payment).

• Do not let your insurance company dictate the quality of dental care that you receive. Your dentist may recommend treatment that is not covered by your insurance policy. If you and the dentist feel that this treatment is needed, have it done. It may cost you some money; however your improved health will be worth the investment.

• When negotiating for dental benefits with your company, request that a dentist review the policy that the insurance company is offering. There are numerous types of policies. A dentist can best ascertain which would be best suited to your needs and desires.

• Insurance companies, large dental groups, and some employers are attempting to decrease company cost for dental insurance. You should be aware of the ramifications of any change in your dental benefits.

• Decrease in the yearly maximum, increase in the deductible scheduled benefit amounts and elimination of certain previously covered items will all decrease the amount of money your company has to pay to insure you. This will also increase the amount of money that you will have to pay the dentist personally.

| Your company may offer you the option of belonging to a: |

Health Maintenance Organization, H.M.O.

This particular type of insurance usually entitles the participant to inexpensive or free dental care.

There is usually one main facility or office for a participating H.M.O. member. The location of this facility *may* be in a convenient location. The insurance company, employer, and you may save some money on the dental care that you receive.

Many H.M.O. facilities hire dentists and pay them flat fees. However, a dentist may work at an H.M.O. for some time and then leave. There is a possibility that you may see several dentists over the course of dental treatment. Also, the location of the H.M.O. may not be convenient to you.

The facility insures large numbers of people. Often a facility is paid a scheduled amount for specific services. This promotes the possibility that your treatment plan may be directed towards the least expensive dental care.

Capitation I.P.A. (Individual Practice Association)

This is a type of H.M.O. where there are several dental care offices as opposed to one main facility. Individual dentists sign up to be a member of this organization and in turn receive the following:

1. An influx of new patients.
2. A guaranteed amount per month for every patient enrolled in this program (whether or not the patient seeks regular dental care).
3 . He or she does not charge the patient any money for any of the covered services that he or she renders.

The insurance company, employer, and you may save some money on the dental care that you receive. Most dentists who sign up for these programs need more patients or want the guaranteed monthly stipend. The financial overtones in this particular system are breeding places for abuse. Dentists can receive money for patients who don't even use their services.

The number of dentists who sign up for these programs varies. By the nature of the contract, you may be forced to see a dentist you find to be unacceptable to your particular situation. Because the dentist is usually not receiving adequate compensation for major dental work, he/she may be inclined to alter your treatment plan accordingly, directing you to a less expensive form of treatment than what you may otherwise need.

P.P.O. (Preferred Provider Organization)

This is known as a closed panel mode of dental care. The employer or insurance company solicit dentists to perform dental care for their employees.

The dentist will receive a large influx of new patients. For this new influx of patients, the dentist will usually discount the fees for company employees. He/she will usually accept the insurance payment as full payment for the services rendered to the patient. This leads to decreased employer cost for dental care benefits. The employee can go to one of the dentists on the list (a preferred provider). If they go there, they usually will not have to pay much for their dental care. They can also go to someone who is not on their list. In that case he/she will usually have to pay for a percentage of his or her dental bills. The dentist who is not on the list will usually not accept the reduced fees for his or her services.

The insurance company, employer, and you may save some money on the dental care that you receive, but your favorite dentist may not be on the list. You may be inclined to change dentists for financial reasons only.

The dentists who sign up for these programs are usually large groups, or private practitioners. For one reason or another, they need more patients. Large groups are often staffed by transient dentists, like H.M.O.'s, which means that the quality of care that you receive may not be consistent. Because of the reduced fees that the dentist receives for doing your dentistry, he/she may be inclined to alter your specific treatment plan. Again, the dental care may be directed towards a less expensive treatment which may not be appropriate for your situation.

Regular Care Insurance

This dental coverage varies with each particular insurance company and each particular insurance policy.

You have the option of seeing the dentist of your choice. You pay a portion of the dental bill. The dentist performs his or her treatments without discounting his or her fees. The treatment plans that he or she presents will usually be directed towards the best dental treatment as opposed to the least expensive care.

Personal Note

I regard any form of dental insurance plan as a potential asset for the patient, dentist, and employer.

Most dental insurance policies will:

1. Lessen the cost of dental care for the patient.
2. Increase the dentist's patient flow.
3. Increase the patient's acceptance of quality dental care.
4. Improve the health of an employer's workforce.

Beware of falling into the dental insurance trap.

Unfortunately, sometimes the insurance plans will interfere with quality of dental care necessary for an individual. Do not let the insurance plan dictate the type of treatment available for you and your family. If dental care costs more than what your plan or company is willing to pay, pay the difference yourself. You will reap the rewards of excellent dental health.

CHAPTER 27

The Future of Dentistry as I See It

"The mind of man is capable of anything because everything is in it, all the past as well as all the future".
Joseph Conrad 1902

Our children and grandchildren will not be burdened by dental disease. Most of the treatment rendered by the dentist will be preventive. Fear and discomfort will be non existent where dental treatment is concerned.

- Educated parents will perform basic dental home-care techniques with their children. This will aid in the prevention of dental breakdown.
- Children will see the dentist early in life, (2-3 years old) and will relate positively to their dentists.
- Dental problems will be detected early and be easily treated.
- Orthodontics will be utilized more often to properly align the dentition for better function. The proper aligning of the teeth will also help to prevent periodontal disease and decay from occurring later in life.
- Future home care will focus more and more on the pre–brushing rinses which were launched in the 1980's as the first in an entirely new category of home care products.

Advanced technology will include:
- Electronic devices such as X-ray machines and light beams, will be able to detect decay before any major destruction has occurred.
- Drills that **do not** make any noise will be created.
- Chemicals, lasers, and new materials might eliminate the need for drilling and filling when cavities are detected early.

- Anti-cavity and anti-periodontal drugs might eliminate the bacteria which cause the destruction of the teeth and gums.
- For individuals needing fillings and crowns, the new restorative materials will last longer and look better than the previous materials.
- The dentist will become an integral part of the medical team in the treatment of headaches through proper diagnosis and treatment of T.M.J. pain and dysfunction.
- Electrical anesthesia or electrical pre-anesthesia will make the virtually painless needle completely painless. Anesthesia will be complete and discomfort during dental treatment will be nonexistent.
- Implants will be used routinely for reconstructing debilitated mouths.
- The profession of dentistry will be the most enjoyable of the medical profession.

CHAPTER 29

Dental Glossary

"The only reason a person gives up a study or becomes confused or unable to learn is because he or she has gone past a word that was not understood."

L. Ron Hubbard

If you are having dental work done, you should be aware of what the dentist is doing. He or she will usually speak to his or her assistant in his or her normal dental vocabulary. There is no reason why you should feel like a foreigner in your own mouth. Learn the dental language.

Briefly review the following major dental terms before your next visit. You and your dentist will be glad you did.

Acrylic - plastic-like material.

Abscess - infection of tooth or gums.

Alveolar - bone surrounding the root of a tooth.

Amalgam - metal combination used to fill teeth.

Analgesics - medications for pain relief.

Anemia - blood disease.

Anesthesia -

1. *Topical:* pain perception elimination on surface tissue.
2. *Local:* pain perception elimination in one area.
3. *General:* pain perception elimination of the entire body.

Anomalies - irregularities.

Antibiotics - medications used to eliminate infections.

Anxiety - a self-inflicted feeling of tension.

Apthous - ulcer, sore.

Attrition - wear on teeth caused by grinding.

Bicuspid - teeth used for tearing. The fourth and fifth teeth from the center.

Bell's Palsy - disruption of the facial nerve.

Bruxism - grinding of the teeth during sleep.

Buccal - near the cheeks.

Calculas - hardened plaque.

Cancer - destructive disease.

Canker sore - viral irritation lasting 7 to 10 days.

Caries - cavities; decay.

Cavity - the part of a tooth that has been destroyed by demineralization.

Cementum - the outer coating of the root of the tooth.

Centric occlusion - the relationship of the upper and lower teeth when fully closed.

Centric relation - the relationship of the upper and lower jaws.

Cleft Palate - an opening in the roof of the mouth.

Crown - the part of the tooth that is visible above the gums.

Crown (cap) - reparative covering placed over a damaged tooth.

Curettage - cleaning of the gum tissue.

Cuspid - the 'eye' tooth. The prominent tooth that is the third tooth from the center.

Cyst - encapsulated defective lesion.

Dentist - a nice guy who cares for, and helps *you* care for your oral health.

Dental floss - string that is used to clean between the teeth.

Dentin - the layer of the tooth between the enamel and pulp.

Denture - artificial replacement teeth.

Diagnosis - evaluation of a problem.

Diastema - a space, usually between the two front teeth.

Disclosing solution - a dye which stains plaque and allows you to see where you missed brushing and flossing.

Edentulous - without teeth.

Enamel - the hard white outer coating of a tooth.

Endodontic Therapy (root canal therapy) - removal of the dead or dying pulp tissue in order to save a tooth.

Explorer - an instrument used to find cavities.

Fluoride - a mineral that adds to tooth strength and helps prevent tooth decay.

Frenum - muscular tissue connecting the lips and gums.

Fracture - break in the tooth or bone.

Gagging - an annoying reflex action.

Gingiva - gum tissue.

Gingival crevice - the area between the tooth and gums.

Gingival recession - the shrinking or diminishing of gum tissue.

Gingivectomy - surgical removal of gum tissue.

Gingivitis - an early stage of gum disease.

Hperplasia - excessive amount of tissue.

Impacted teeth - teeth which can be found under the gums or bone.

Impressions - imprints of the dental arch.

Incisors - the front cutting teeth.

Inflammation - the body's response to an irritant.

Infection - Bacterial or viral disruption of bodily tissue.

Jaws - The bony support for the chewing apparatus.

Labial - lips.

Lingual - tongue.

Lymph nodes - areas to which infections can drain.

Malocclusion - misalignment of the teeth.

Mandible - lower jaw.

Mastication - chewing.

Maxilla - upper jaw.

Molar - large posterior tooth used for chewing.

Mouth - an incredibly important and complex body structure.

Needle - not nearly as terrible as you might mentally perceive it to be.

Nerves - lines of communication between bodily parts and the brain.

Nervousness - a feeling that some people get when they see a dentist.

Occlusion - the way in which the teeth come together.

Odontogenesis imperfecta - poorly developed teeth.

Operative dentistry - drilling and filling to repair teeth.

Oral hygiene - proper brushing and flossing.

Oral mucosa - tissue within the mouth.

Orthodontics - a specialty field within the dental profession which is solely related to straightening teeth and correcting malocclusions.

Overbite - a type of malocclusion.

Overjet - a type of malocclusion.

Pain - a thing of the past when modern dental techniques are used.

Palate - the hard area on the roof of the mouth.

Palpate - Examine by touch.

Parasthesia - a numbing sensation caused by damaged nerve tissue. This is usually temporary.

Parotid gland - a saliva producing gland on the inside of the cheek.

Patient - a guest in the dental office.

Penicillin - an antibiotic that helps to eliminate a bacterial infection.

Periapical abscess - infection at the end of the root.

Periodontal abscess - infection of the gum tissue.

Periodontal disease - generalized chronic infection of the gum tissue.

Periodontal pockets - areas around the teeth where infections can start.

Periodontist - Dental specialists who treats periodontal disease.

Periodontitis - early to middle stages of periodontal disease.

Plaque - a white, sticky substance found on un-brushed teeth; a combination of food and bacteria.

Preventive dentistry - treating potential problems to avoid major problems from occurring.

Pre–brushing rinse - an over the counter product used before brushing and flossing to loosen and detach plaque.

Primary dentition - the baby teeth.

Prognathism - protruded lower jaw.

Prognosis - predicted outcome.

Prophylaxis - dental cleaning.

Prosthesis - dental appliance that usually replaces teeth.

Prosthetic dentistry - the art of restoring a destroyed dentition.

Pulp - the innermost portion of the tooth.

Pulpitis - inflamed pulp.

Radiograph - an X-ray picture of the teeth.

Referrals - recommending other patients to visit your dentist.

Resorption - breakdown of the tooth, gums, or bone.

Restorations - fillings, crowns, etc.

Retainer - orthodontic appliance.

Retromolar pad - gum tissue behind the last tooth.

Rheumatic fever - childhood disease which can cause heart complications and potential problems with dental treatment.

Root - the portion of the tooth that is firmly embedded in the jaw bone.

Root canal (endodontics) - removal of dead or dying pulp tissue to save the tooth.

Saliva - oral fluid.

Salivary glands - producers of oral fluid called saliva.

Sinus - air spaces in the maxilla bone.

Sinusitis - infection of these air spaces.

Smoking - an unnecessary habit which can be very destructive.

Study casts - models of the dental arches.

Surgery - a procedure sometimes necessary to remove teeth and repair gum tissue.

Temporomandibular joint (T.M.J.) - a complicated joint that allows the lower jaw freedom of movement for chewing.

T.M.J. (pain dysfunction syndrome) - pain and dysfunction caused by an overworked temporomandiblular joint.

Tongue - a muscular structure in the mouth that is used for speech and chewing.

Tooth - one of 32 precious oral possessions.

Torus - extra bone in the palate or inner portion of the lower jaw.

Treatment plan - an organized approach to solve your particular dental problem.

Trigeminal nerve - a main nerve trunk of the oral-facial complex.

Xerostomia - dry mouth.

X-rays - pictures.

For additional copies of this book,
please contact our office.
Dr. Robert S. Rauch
91 Cherry Street, Milford, CT 06460
(203) 874-5577